# Praise for *We Deserve More*

"*We Deserve More* truly captures how medical care can retraumatize us when compassion and consent are missing. Survivors already carry a lasting trauma; we deserve better care."

—**Hadley Duvall,** *survivor and activist*

"Bigger than any single billing practice, restrictive policy, or abortion ban, Nikki puts words to a truth rarely expressed: Something is deeply wrong with the way reproductive healthcare is provided—or rather, not provided—in this country. But far from bemoan the inevitable, this books provides the tools each of us can use to begin remaking a healthcare system that actually cares for women and pregnant people."

—**Molly Duane,** *JD, MPH, litigation director of Amplify Legal, Formerly of the Center for Reproductive Rights*

"From over a decade of clinical experience as an OB-GYN Physician Assistant, Nikki Sapiro Vinckier paints us a picture we cannot look away from—describing just how broken our reproductive health system is and the daily harms that system enacts on both patients and providers. Importantly, she compels us to go beyond anger and step into action, with concrete strategies to reshape and retake our reproductive health care into our own hands."

—**Latona Giwa,** *executive director, Repro TLC*

"*We Deserve More* is the book I wish I had read decades ago. It should be on the reading list for every book club. It should be part of the curriculum for every Women and Gender's Studies program. It should be required reading for every medical student. This is the book I will gift to my friends (male and female). This is a book for people who give a damn about women."

—**Kristin Cravens Hutton,** *@kris.and.dave*

"The fight over reproductive healthcare is deeply personal, and all of us, men included, have a stake in whether or not people have access to the care they need. This book provides a comprehensive guide for navigating a system that creates endless barriers to that essential care, including how men like us can fully support the women in our life navigating those barriers on a daily basis."
   —**Oren Jacobson,** *Men4Choice founder and senior advisor*

"In *We Deserve More*, Nikki Sapiro Vinckier uses her experience as a clinician within the reproductive healthcare system to help patients effectively navigate it. It is a wonderful resource for anyone seeking support through the complexities of provider relationships, insurance frustrations, online misinformation, and much more."
   —**Becca Rea-Tucker,** *author of* The Abortion Companion: An Affirming Handbook for Your Choice and Your Journey *(2026)*

# We Deserve More

# We Deserve More

*Why Reproductive Healthcare Is Broken*
And What You Can Do About It

Nikki Sapiro Vinckier, PA-C

**JOSSEY-BASS**
A Wiley Brand

Copyright © 2026 by Nikki Sapiro Vinckier. All rights reserved.

Published by John Wiley & Sons, Inc., Hoboken, New Jersey.

No part of this publication may be reproduced, stored in a retrieval system, or transmitted in any form or by any means, electronic, mechanical, photocopying, recording, scanning, or otherwise, except as permitted under Section 107 or 108 of the 1976 United States Copyright Act, without either the prior written permission of the Publisher, or authorization through payment of the appropriate per-copy fee to the Copyright Clearance Center, Inc., 222 Rosewood Drive, Danvers, MA 01923, (978) 750-8400, fax (978) 750-4470, or on the web at www.copyright.com. Requests to the Publisher for permission should be addressed to the Permissions Department, John Wiley & Sons, Inc., 111 River Street, Hoboken, NJ 07030, (201) 748-6011, fax (201) 748-6008, or online at http://www.wiley.com/go/permission.

The manufacturer's authorized representative according to the EU General Product Safety Regulation is Wiley-VCH GmbH, Boschstr. 12, 69469 Weinheim, Germany, e-mail: Product_Safety@wiley.com.

**Trademarks:** Wiley and the Wiley logo are trademarks or registered trademarks of John Wiley & Sons, Inc. and/or its affiliates in the United States and other countries and may not be used without written permission. All other trademarks are the property of their respective owners. John Wiley & Sons, Inc. is not associated with any product or vendor mentioned in this book.

**Limit of Liability/Disclaimer of Warranty:** While the publisher and the authors have used their best efforts in preparing this work, including a review of the content of the work, neither the publisher nor the authors make any representations or warranties with respect to the accuracy or completeness of the contents of this work and specifically disclaim all warranties, including without limitation any implied warranties of merchantability or fitness for a particular purpose. No warranty may be created or extended by sales representatives, written sales materials or promotional statements for this work. The fact that an organization, website, or product is referred to in this work as a citation and/or potential source of further information does not mean that the publisher and authors endorse the information or services the organization, website, or product may provide or recommendations it may make. This work is sold with the understanding that the publisher is not engaged in rendering professional services. The advice and strategies contained herein may not be suitable for your situation. You should consult with a specialist where appropriate. Further, readers should be aware that websites listed in this work may have changed or disappeared between when this work was written and when it is read. Neither the publisher nor authors shall be liable for any loss of profit or any other commercial damages, including but not limited to special, incidental, consequential, or other damages.

For general information on our other products and services, please contact our Customer Care Department within the United States at (800) 762-2974, outside the United States at (317) 572- 3993 or fax (317) 572-4002. For product technical support, you can find answers to frequently asked questions or reach us via live chat at https://support.wiley.com.

If you believe you've found a mistake in this book, please bring it to our attention by emailing our reader support team at wileysupport@wiley.com with the subject line "Possible Book Errata Submission."

Wiley also publishes its books in a variety of electronic formats. Some content that appears in print may not be available in electronic formats. For more information about Wiley products, visit our web site at www.wiley.com.

*Library of Congress Cataloging-in-Publication Data is Available:*

ISBN: 9781394407798 (Cloth)
ISBN: 9781394407804 (ePub)
ISBN: 9781394407811 (ePDF)

Cover Design: Wiley
Cover Image: © cnythzl/Getty Images
SKY10150491_032426

This book is dedicated to every person who's
ever sat in an exam room, scared to speak up.
To the ones who were dismissed,
doubted, or left with more questions than answers.

To those who Googled after. Who didn't go back.
Who still carry the weight of care that fell short.

To the ones who stayed quiet
and to the ones who couldn't anymore.
To the patients who became advocates.
To the advocates who were told they were too loud.
To the clinicians trying to do better inside a broken system.
And to everyone just trying to be heard.

To my best friend, Ashley,
who let me in during her hardest moments,
making it achingly clear that this book was beyond needed.

To my husband, Mark,
who is an example that men can be a part of the solution.

To my daughter,
who will one day walk into this same system.
May it be softer by then.
May she walk in ready. May they listen.
May she know she deserves more.

This book is for all of us.
You deserve more.
We deserve more.

# Contents

About the Author   xiii
Preface   xv
Introduction   xix

**Part One: What's Wrong with the System**   1

**Chapter 1:** The Roots of a Broken System   3
How History Shaped the Care We Get and Why It Still Fails Us Now

**Chapter 2:** How the Limits of OB-GYN Training Lead to Gaps in Care   9
From What's Taught to What You Experience—How Training Gaps Become Care Gaps

**Chapter 3:** Missing Pieces, Missing Care   35
When Silence, Stigma, and Neglect Leave Patients "Unseen"

**Chapter 4:** Care Wasn't Built for Everyone   67
Some People Aren't Just Falling Through the Cracks, They've Been Failed from the Beginning

| | | |
|---|---|---|
| Chapter 5: | The Illusion of Coverage | 87 |
| | How Insurance Turns Access into an Obstacle Course | |
| Chapter 6: | Broken System, Good People | 105 |
| | Not All Providers Are Bad, but They're Working in a System That Makes It Hard to be Good | |
| Chapter 7: | The Trauma We Carry In | 123 |
| | When the System Doesn't See Trauma, It Risks Creating More of It | |

## Part Two: When the System Gets Personal — 149

| | | |
|---|---|---|
| Chapter 8: | When Culture Illuminates the Failures | 151 |
| | How Stories Shatter Silence, Build Community, and Push Medicine to Pay Attention | |
| Chapter 9: | Too Little Time | 161 |
| | Why Short Visits Leave Patients Feeling Unseen and How to Reclaim Your Voice When the Clock Is Against You | |
| Chapter 10: | The Algorithm Will See You Now | 175 |
| | How Social Media Is Shaping the Way We Seek, Share, and Trust Health Information | |
| Chapter 11: | When Your Voice Isn't Enough: Gaslighting, Bias, and Discrimination in Care | 193 |
| | The Systemic Failures That Silence Patients and the Tools You Need to be Heard | |

## Part Three: Your Body, Your Voice — 207

| | | |
|---|---|---|
| Chapter 12: | Learning Your Body and Your Needs | 209 |
| | You Can't Advocate for Yourself if You've Been Taught to Ignore Your Body; Let's Change That | |
| Chapter 13: | Finding Care That Sees You | 219 |
| | Because the Right Provider Doesn't Just Treat Your Body. They Respect Your Whole Self | |

## Contents

**Chapter 14:** How to Get Ready, Speak Up, and Handle What Comes    235
    Speaking Up Is Power; Knowing What to Do When You're Dismissed Is Protection

**Chapter 15:** Asking for Pain Management    245
    You Shouldn't Have to Suffer Through It, but You Do Need to Ask Ahead of Time

**Chapter 16:** Care Beyond the Exam Room    257
    Self-Care Isn't Separate from Healthcare, It's Part of It

**Chapter 17:** Lessons from Abroad    267
    How Global Models Reveal What's Possible, and How to Bring Those Lessons Home

**Chapter 18:** This Isn't Extra; This Is Your Right    281
    How to Take Everything You've Learned and Use It to Get the Care You Deserve

## Additional Content

References    301

Before we get going, I want to take a quick moment to ask you to check your voter registration or register to vote. It takes just a few minutes, and it matters more than most of us realize.

Voting is part of your civic health. It is also part of your reproductive health. The policies that shape access to contraception, abortion care, IVF, maternal health services, and insurance coverage are decided by people we elect at every level. Showing up at the ballot box is one way we protect our bodies, our families, and our communities.

I've included a QR code here to make it easy.

Take a second, scan it, and make sure your voice is ready for the next election.

# About the Author

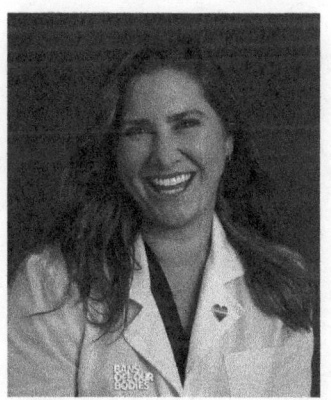

**Nikki Sapiro Vinckier, PA-C (she/her),** is an OB-GYN Physician Associate, reproductive rights advocate and educator, digital creator, and founder of Take Back Trust, a patient-centered education and empowerment platform helping people navigate reproductive healthcare with clarity and confidence. She has spent over a decade in clinical practice and works at the intersection of medicine, media, and movement to advance reproductive health literacy and patient autonomy.

Through videos, guides, op-eds, and national campaigns reaching millions each month, Nikki translates complex reproductive health issues into accessible, actionable information. Her work is grounded in real-world patient care and shaped by the realities clinicians and patients face inside a system that often fails them. She is known for pairing clinical accuracy with unapologetic advocacy, relentlessly calling out systemic barriers while defending patient autonomy.

A California native now based in Michigan, Nikki is a proud mom of three kids, along with a rescue dog and cat. She believes deeply in healthcare that is honest, inclusive, and affirming. *We Deserve More* and *We Deserve More: The Workbook* are her debut books.

You can find her on all platforms as @nikkivinck.

# Preface

I never thought I'd write a book. I thought my work would always stay within the clinic walls. One patient, one story, one exam room at a time. But outside those walls, the same stories kept chasing me. I'd open my phone and see them everywhere: women talking about the years it took to get an endometriosis diagnosis. A reel about how painful an IUD insertion was. Someone crying in their car after yet another appointment where their pain was brushed off. Hundreds of comments echoing the same refrain.

Different people. Different symptoms. Different cities. Some living with daily pain so intense it reshapes their lives. Others calling out of work every month because of an unmanageable flow. Some simply knowing that once they hit 40, something shifted in their body and no one seems to have answers. Every age. Every race. Every income level. Every stage of life.

And yet, when you strip away the details, the stories collapse into the same core truth: *I'm not being heard. I'm not being believed. I'm not getting the help I need.*

These aren't bad-luck, one-off, or isolated experiences. This is happening every single day, in every part of the United States. I keep hearing it: from patients after weeding through doctors, hoping the next one might finally take them seriously. From friends texting me questions their doctor either ignored or didn't have time to answer. And, honestly, I've felt it myself, through my own reproductive healthcare needs and in the births of my three children within this same system.

For a decade, I sat in exam rooms seeing 20 to 25 patients a day, watching the system grind down both patients and providers. I was frustrated, but more than that, I was determined to be different. To be the one who listened. The one who made patients feel seen, supported, cared for.

As it became apparent that *Roe v. Wade* was going to fall I started getting more involved in advocacy work as well. I participated in and lead multiple reproductive health roundtables across our state discussing the implications of the political warfare raging over women's bodies. I gathered thousands of signatures for our ballot proposal to add reproductive freedom to our state constitution and I fundraised for our local abortion fund.

I wore my pride pin on my white coat. I brought up voting, not partisan politics. After all, both the American Medical Association and American College of Obstetricians and Gynecologists remind us that civic health and medical health are inseparable, and access to the ballot is directly related to access to care.

In fall 2024 I was told to take my pin off, that it was "too polarizing," and told voting was never appropriate to discuss. And just a few days later I was fired. Officially, I was told that I wasn't a "professional fit." The truth? I didn't *fit* into the small box they wanted me to stay in, which was to follow suit. To stand in line. To fit the mold. Their mold. Don't challenge. Be obedient. As an advanced practice provider, I was supposed to be a physician extender, not a physician challenger. My role was to make their lives easier, not raise uncomfortable questions or advocate for change. But watching the way care was delivered, what was said, what was ignored, didn't sit well with me.

Because the model only serves patients who have no complicated health needs, never deal with pain, don't live in a larger body, can answer all necessary questions in an eight-minute slot, never have to scramble for childcare or beg for time off to make a 1 p.m. appointment, have flawless insurance, ample cash when things aren't covered, and check the normative boxes of being straight and white.

As women, we're told: don't be too loud, too bold, too strong. Don't ask for too much. We're asked to shrink ourselves to fit into the box instead of being given the tools and support to bust it open and build a whole new one. When I lost my job, I realized that if the system didn't want my voice inside the clinic, I'd carry it everywhere else.

Stepping back from day-to-day clinical work gave me what I think of as the 20,000-foot view: I could see why a clinician might feel boxed in by liability, time, guidelines, or billing codes, *and* why a patient walks away feeling dismissed, frustrated, or unheard. I understood that the tension between providers and patients isn't usually about either side failing; it's about a system designed in a way that makes collision inevitable.

Clinicians are trained to stay within strict guardrails, document in specific ways, and keep visits short. Patients, meanwhile, show up with layered histories, real fears, and needs that rarely fit neatly into a 10-minute slot. When those realities crash into each other, it can feel deeply personal, but often, it's systemic. Seeing that clearly made me realize just how important it is to name those forces, and how urgent the need is to equip patients tools to navigate them. So I set out to write this book.

I started learning about the system itself. About who gets left behind. About the people who walk out of appointments feeling invisible, the ones who turn to the internet because their doctor didn't have the time or space for them. I started paying attention to the rise of social media influencers and movements stepping in to fill the void. I emersed myself in conversations happening behind the scenes with clinicians who, like me, felt trapped by the constraints of the system.

I want this book to show is that reproductive healthcare reflects how we see each other as fully human, and whether our healthcare system is willing to treat us women that way. (After all, nothing about men's bodies is made political.) But, for the record, this whole book will be written from a nonpartisan lens. Reproductive healthcare shouldn't be political. It's about basic human dignity. It's about whether someone can access safe, timely, compassionate care when they need it most. It's a matter of health, safety, and survival. It is universal. It touches every community, every family, every identity. It shapes the lives of women, men, and trans and nonbinary people. It touches parents, those who want to be parents one day and those who never want kids at all.

I'll be completely honest: some of the things we hope for in healthcare just aren't realistic right now. Unfortunately the system isn't built to give you the level of understanding, support, and compassion you deserve. But I firmly believe that if you want better care, the first step is knowing what you're up against. That means learning not just about your body but also about the system itself. So let's jump in.

# Introduction

There are books that will teach you all about reproductive healthcare: how your uterus works, what causes cramps, and how to manage menopause. There are books that will guide you on your fertility journey and ones that will tell you what to expect when pregnant.

This isn't that book.

This isn't a biology textbook. It's a lesson. Then a road map and a lifeline. It is a guide to help you understand and navigate a system that was never built to fully support you, and too often leaves you feeling confused, dismissed, or on your own.

And before we go further, I want to be clear about who I am. I'm not a doctor. I'm a physician associate (PA). If you aren't familiar with PAs, we're licensed medical professionals who complete an intensive two- to three-year graduate program and are trained to diagnose, treat, prescribe, and care for patients, usually in close partnership with physicians. I chose this path because it allowed me more time with patients, more freedom to focus on education and conversation, and a career built on collaboration. I didn't become a PA as a fallback or consolation prize.

Working as an OB-GYN PA for over a decade has given me a rare vantage point. I've been close enough to the physician training model to understand how it works, but with enough distance to ask why it so often fails the very people it's meant to serve. I've watched medicine at its best, and I've watched it falter. The gaps are real. And together, we can start patching them.

I now find myself outside the clinic, doing reproductive health advocacy and creating digital content. The same questions I once heard in exam rooms now pour into my inbox and comment sections. People are desperate for reproductive healthcare information that feels clear, trustworthy, and practical. They are looking for education that meets them where they are, not buried in jargon or hidden behind closed doors. Showing up online has revealed just how deep that hunger runs, and how powerful it can be to give people the language, context, and tools they can carry into real life.

The truth is the system is flawed. Truly flawed. But I'm not here to redesign the system from the top down. There are others qualified to reinvent medical training, overhaul reimbursement models, or rebuild healthcare policy. That's not my forte, nor is it the purpose of this book.

This book holds both truths at once:

The system is broken.
And you still deserve good care.

And the fact that good care feels like luck? That's the problem.

This book is about pulling back the curtain so you can finally see *why*. Why doctors' training emphasizes emergencies over everyday realities. Why insurance companies can dictate more about your care than your provider does. Why visits are rushed, why trust keeps breaking down, and why so many of us end up searching the internet for the answers we should've gotten in the exam room.

This is a guide to understanding and navigating reproductive healthcare in America today. It comes from my vantage point, built from what I saw every single day in the clinic, then shaped by my own experiences and having had three children within this same system. It has been further honed by the journeys I've walked alongside friends through miscarriages, birth control battles, fertility treatments, hysterectomies, and menopause. These stories stretch across every corner of the United States and touch upon every moment in reproductive healthcare.

It's what I see every time I open my social media feed. And it's what I've heard from thousands of patients. People who have been told "everything looks fine" when nothing about their life felt fine. People who arrived in my exam room carrying years of unanswered questions and unaddressed pain.

This book is my way of sharing what I've learned: a way to name what's happening, to understand why so many of us aren't getting what we need from the system right now, and to see how we got here. Until the day the system changes, it's also a way to map out where we go from here.

Because naming the problem isn't enough. You need a plan. In these pages you'll feel seen and validated. You may feel anger and rage. But my goal is that these pages also give you a glimmer of hope. That they give you the practical tools: questions to ask, scripts to lean on, and strategies to carry into the moments that matter most. You'll learn what to expect, how to prepare, and what your real options are.

In Part One, we'll dig into what's wrong with the system itself. From the classroom to the clinic, you'll see how blind spots in training, gaps in insurance, and systemic bias create the conditions that make care feel rushed and impersonal.

Part Two traces what happens when those flaws get personal, when they show up as misdiagnosis, silence, grief, gaslighting, cultural erasure, and growing mistrust. This is where the consequences land in real life, in real bodies.

And Part Three is where the power shifts back to you. It's the road map: the strategies, scripts, and mindset shifts that can help you walk into appointments prepared, steady your voice when you're dismissed, and navigate a system that was never built with you in mind.

Healthcare in America is broken. I wish we could burn it all down, start fresh, and build the care system we actually deserve. I wish we could take lessons from other parts of the world, places where systems are built to serve people, not wear them down. Since we can't, we have to learn how to navigate the one we've got, and how to make it work for you.

But here's the truth: we are in the middle of an awakening. A reckoning. A moment where women have realized just how long we've been silenced. Silenced about our pain, our choices, our bodies, about too many damn things that shape our lives. An awakening to the fact that men have sat at the tables deciding our health without us for too damn long.

This book is part of that awakening. Part of that reckoning. It's here to name what has been ignored, to give language to what's been silenced, and to hand you the tools to take back power, in the exam room and far beyond it.

Because you deserve more.

**We deserve more.**

**One more quick note before we dive in:** Though I am a clinician, I'm not here as *your* clinician. This book isn't medical advice, it's education, context, and tools. My goal is to give you language to use in the exam room, strategies to navigate the system, and questions to help you advocate for yourself. Every body is different, every situation is unique, and your medical decisions should always be made with a qualified professional you trust.

**A note for clinicians:** If you're reading this as a healthcare provider, thank you and I'm glad you're here. You've probably felt these limits pressing in on you, too. The rushed visits, the impossible demands, the frustration of wanting to give more when the system won't let you. At the end of this book there's an addendum made just for you, a way forward, even inside a broken system. Because your role matters, your impact matters, and small changes from inside the walls of medicine can make a difference.

# Part One

# WHAT'S WRONG WITH THE SYSTEM

*Before We Can Talk About How to Get Better Care,
We Have to Learn What's Broken*

Part One pulls back the curtain on the medical system that so many of us have come to fear, mistrust, or avoid altogether. It names the harmful and often hidden history of gynecology. A history built on experimentation without consent, racism, and systemic abuse. It examines some of the gaping holes in medical training for obstetrician-gynecologists (OB-GYNs). It explains some of the reasons why your visits feel rushed, why care feels impersonal, and why getting help can feel like a fight. It explores how insurance dictates what gets done, what gets covered, and who gets seen. It shares that most providers are good people with good intentions stuck in a system that doesn't allow for great care. And then it confronts the invisible weight that too many of us carry into these rooms: trauma, shame, and memories of being dismissed.

If you've ever walked out of an appointment feeling confused, hurt, or dehumanized, this is where you'll start to understand why.

But this isn't just a takedown. It's a translation. Part One focuses on helping you see the system for what it is. It helps you understand how everything fits together so you can move through your care with more clarity and confidence.

# Chapter 1

# The Roots of a Broken System

*How History Shaped the Care We Get and Why It Still Fails Us Now*

Reproductive healthcare didn't break overnight. The system you walk into every time you step into a doctor's office wasn't born last year or even last decade. It's the product of centuries of change, layer on layer, that built the landscape we live with today.

In its earliest forms, reproductive care was community-based. Birth, miscarriage, fertility, and menopause were life events managed at home, surrounded by people who had lived through them, too. Midwives, healers, and women caring for women carried the knowledge. It wasn't perfect, but it was personal. Care was relational, not transactional. Trust came from shared experience, community, and continuity.

That began to shift once medicine professionalized. As universities and hospitals consolidated power, lived experience was devalued and credentialed expertise became the new currency of care. Midwives, who had long been trusted guides in their communities, were increasingly sidelined. In some cases midwives were criminalized as physicians (predominantly white men) claimed formal control over birth and women's health. What had been rooted in kinship and trust was redefined inside institutions. And with that shift came a rupture: the continuity that once defined reproductive care gave way to hierarchy, surveillance, and medical dominance.

The erasure hit hardest in communities of color. Before the Civil War, roughly half of all midwives in the United States were Black. These midwives anchored care across the rural South. They weren't just catching babies. They were providing prenatal care, postpartum support, contraception, and even abortion at a time when Black women had almost no other way to control their bodies. They held communities together when families were torn apart by slavery, and they kept records, traditions, and networks alive. But as childbirth moved into hospitals in the early twentieth century, Black midwives were targeted. Physicians smeared them as dirty or ignorant, lawmakers piled on restrictions, and training programs shut them out. Indigenous midwives faced similar suppression, as colonial policies and medical authorities sought to replace community-based practices with hospital-controlled care. By mid-century, midwives attended only a small fraction of births in the United States, even though studies showed maternal deaths were often *lower* in areas with more midwife involvement.

This wasn't just a story of "progress." It was a story of power. Knowledge rooted in African American, Indigenous, and immigrant traditions was dismissed as illegitimate, while elite, white, male medicine wrote itself in as the authority. The move to formalize and centralize care created a narrower, more hierarchical system. A structure that cut off communities from the care traditions that had served them for centuries.

The echoes of that shift are still with us today. When people say they don't trust medical institutions, especially concerning birth, that mistrust isn't new. It goes back to the moment care was pulled out of communities' hands and rebuilt inside a system that was never designed to include everyone's voice.

## The Dark Origins of Gynecology

Modern gynecology was built on the suffering of Black women. Dr. J. Marion Sims, often referred to as the "father of gynecology," perfected his surgical techniques by operating on enslaved women. Without anesthesia, without consent, and without believing their pain was real.

There were many women who remain anonymous, but we know the names of three women: Anarcha, Lucy, and Betsy. Anarcha was 17 when Sims started cutting into her. Thirty surgeries over four years. Thirty. She was held down by other enslaved women while this man experimented on her body. He was convinced that Black women didn't feel pain the way white women did. Lucy and Betsey suffered alongside her, their names barely remembered, their agony dismissed as the necessary cost of medical progress.

This is the foundation of modern gynecology and a significant thread in the history of obstetrics and sexual health. The precedent of experimentation without regard to pain. The concept that some bodies matter and others don't. That some people deserve care and others deserve to be used.

The pattern didn't stop there. From 1932 to 1972, the US government conducted what became known as the Tuskegee Study. Essentially watching Black men die of syphilis even after penicillin was discovered. They told these men they were getting free healthcare for "bad blood." They were actually being studied like lab rats while a curable disease ate away at their bodies and minds. Forty years of an insanely harmful and deadly study. Decades of doctors trained during an era when medical racism wasn't hidden, it was common practice.

Meanwhile, women were being used as test subjects for drugs that companies knew could be dangerous. Pregnant women got thalidomide for morning sickness without being told it could cause birth defects. When thousands of babies were born without limbs, the response wasn't accountability, it was damage control. The Dalkon Shield intrauterine device infected, sterilized, and killed women and the company hid the data. Henrietta Lacks had her cells stolen and used to build billion-dollar medical breakthroughs while her family couldn't afford health insurance. Over and over, the message was clear: bodies (specifically female bodies and Black bodies) are for using, not caring for.

And the dark history isn't just confined to the United States. After World War II, the Nuremberg Trials exposed horrific, nonconsensual medical experiments conducted by Nazi physicians on Jewish prisoners during the Holocaust. Those proceedings gave birth to the Nuremberg Code, which insisted on voluntary consent, minimizing suffering, and ensuring that medical research benefits society. For reproductive healthcare, the lessons were direct: informed consent and patient autonomy must be the cornerstone of ethical care. The code is a reminder, born out of atrocities, that medicine without consent is not medicine at all.

Here's what makes this all particularly maddening: most providers today have no idea these things happened. Medical schools don't teach it. This isn't just an oversight. When you don't teach the history of medical racism, you don't have to deal with its ongoing effects. When providers don't understand why communities might be suspicious of medical recommendations, they see skepticism as "noncompliance" instead of justified caution. And when providers don't learn this history, they can't recognize the ways it still shapes disparities in pain management, maternal mortality, and reproductive autonomy today.

## When Medicine Became About Emergencies

For most of history, reproductive care was a matter of survival. Hemorrhage, infection, and eclampsia turned pregnancy and childbirth into some of the most dangerous events in a woman's life. Hospitals and physicians had one mission: keep women alive through delivery. Crisis care was the measure of success because maternal mortality was devastatingly common.

That focus saved lives. But when antibiotics, anesthesia, blood banks, and surgical advances dramatically reduced deaths, the training model and focus didn't evolve. Generations of OB-GYNs were still taught to think like doctors in the 1920s while practicing a century later. They learn to act fast in the face of catastrophe, but not to linger with slower, chronic problems that unfold over years. Their training builds the reflex to run toward alarms, not to sit patiently with complexity.

The merger was driven by hospitals and medical schools that wanted administrative efficiency, not by patient needs or evidence that the fields belonged together. On paper, it streamlined departments. In practice, it streamlined women's lives into pregnancy, birth, and emergencies. Everything else—contraception, painful sex, menopause, ongoing pelvic pain—was treated as secondary, optional, or not worth addressing at all.

That merger left the field with an identity crisis. OB-GYN became the catch-all for every issue involving a uterus: pregnancy, Pap smears, irregular bleeding, infertility, pregnancy loss, contraception counseling, and perimenopause. But the specialty's training remained crisis-driven. Residents spend months delivering babies, managing hemorrhages, and rushing into emergency surgeries. What they spend far less time on is just as telling: counseling someone through perimenopause, addressing sexual pain, or helping a patient manage chronic pelvic symptoms.

The fallout is real. OB-GYNs are trained to stop a hemorrhage in seconds, but many never had structured training on how to respond when someone says their periods are wrecking their quality of life. They learn to deliver a baby safely, but not necessarily how to support the fatigue, brain fog, or mood shifts that come years later. They can perform a hysterectomy with precision, but may not have been given the tools to guide patients through the subtler transitions of menopause. It isn't about lack of dedication or compassion, it's about a training model designed for emergencies, not the everyday realities that shape patients' lives.

And because medical schools, board exams, and residency programs still prize crisis management above everything else, that imbalance gets reinforced over and over. What isn't life-threatening rarely gets attention. Which is why so many patients today walk away from appointments feeling brushed aside. It's not necessarily about individual providers failing, it's about a system still built for emergencies, not experiences.

## How This History Lives in Your Exam Room Today

This history lives in every syllabus, every residency program, every checklist that defines what counts as medicine. It shows up in the curriculum blueprint. It shows up in the health disparities and in policies that treat reproductive decisions as political battles rather than healthcare. Abortion bans and contraception limits aren't new. Bans echo long traditions of controlling whose bodies mattered. And when providers dismiss your pain, they are often, sometimes unknowingly, repeating that precedent.

The missing piece of change is education. Understanding this history isn't about living in the past, it's about seeing the present clearly. Once you understand the system's design, you stop blaming yourself for its failures. You can begin to navigate differently, with intention, and demand care that meets your needs.

The story isn't over. From here we move from history straight into the heart of OB-GYN training today so you can understand exactly what's missing from your provider's education and what to do about it.

## Chapter 2

# How the Limits of OB-GYN Training Lead to Gaps in Care

*From What's Taught to What You Experience—
How Training Gaps Become Care Gaps*

The previous chapter gave a brief history of reproductive healthcare: the foundations no one likes to talk about and the horrors that shaped the field. Once you are faced with those details, it's hard to unsee them. It's important to know the history in order to understand how the system was built. Then you have more tools to be able to navigate the ways it works today. Because this isn't just about a distant history; it's also about the choices made in the last few decades, and it's about what we're all experiencing right now.

If your gynecologic care has ever felt rushed, incomplete, or disconnected from the reality of your life and your experiences, you're not imagining it. The gaps you feel aren't just echoes of history, they're also baked into how medical training is structured today. And that structure leaves too many needs unmet.

The problems you may have experienced aren't necessarily because your provider didn't care enough. They're the result of a broken system that decides what gets prioritized, what gets skipped, and what never even makes it into the curriculum. Healthcare in America prioritizes procedures over conversational care or bedside manner. From day one, medical education channels future OB-GYNs toward pathology over presence. Procedures over people. Standardization over nuance. Crisis management over quality of life.

We'll talk about medical school, training, residency, and care deserts that shape the experience. We'll talk about research, or the lack thereof. And then we'll talk about what's missing altogether, because when something gets skipped in the classroom, it usually gets skipped in the clinic, too. Silence in the syllabus turns into silence in the exam room. And that silence shows up in your care.

But before we dive into how you can get the care you need, it's worth stepping back and asking a more basic question: is the OB-GYN even the right person to be addressing it?

## The Lack of Primary Care

For more and more patients, their OB-GYN isn't just a reproductive health specialist anymore. They've defaulted to an everything doctor: a point person for blood pressure checks, cholesterol screening, flu shots, depression screening, sleep issues, and whatever else comes up.

That's not how the system was designed. Traditionally, your care would be anchored by a primary care provider (PCP), someone trained to look at the whole health picture, manage chronic conditions, and coordinate with specialists when needed.

In the United States, that usually means one of two types of physicians:

- **Internal medicine (IM):** These doctors specialize in adult medicine, often with deep expertise in managing complex or chronic health conditions like diabetes, hypertension, heart disease, or autoimmune disorders. They can prescribe and manage most forms of basic contraception, perform clinical breast exams, and order mammograms. They *typically* do not perform Pap smears or procedures like intrauterine device insertions. For gynecologic screening and procedures, they'll usually refer you to an OB-GYN or a family medicine provider.
- **Family medicine (FM):** These doctors are trained to care for patients of all ages. They can manage chronic conditions, provide preventive screenings, treat acute illnesses, and offer a more comprehensive range of reproductive healthcare than internal medicine. This often includes Pap smears, contraception counseling and prescriptions, clinical breast exams, and even prenatal care, especially in rural or underserved areas.

Your PCP would refer you to specialists when needed, whether that's a cardiologist for your heart, a dermatologist for your skin, or an OB-GYN for reproductive health concerns that require specialized surgical expertise, complex gynecologic diagnosis, or prenatal care.

For a healthy, nonpregnant person with basic reproductive healthcare needs, a family medicine provider can typically handle everything without the need for a separate OB-GYN. But for anyone with more complex reproductive needs, such as an abnormal Pap, irregular bleeding, or chronic pelvic pain, the ideal setup is usually a PCP plus an OB-GYN.

The problem is that fewer people have a PCP at all. Access is shrinking, wait times are growing, and for many, especially in rural areas, it feels easier to just rely on the provider they already see for their Pap smear or birth control refill. And so, OB-GYNs have become de facto primary care providers for millions of patients all across America.

But here's the issue: OB-GYN training isn't built to replace primary care. Their residency is designed to make them surgical experts and reproductive health specialists, not comprehensive primary care physicians.

This mismatch leaves gaps. If you're only seeing your OB-GYN, you might be missing critical screenings. Colon cancer screening, skin checks, and bone density scans often fall outside their usual scope. You might not get consistent management of chronic conditions. And because OB-GYN visits are already crammed with reproductive priorities, there's even less time to explore non-gynecologic concerns during visits.

## The Impossible Scope of OB-GYN Care

This mismatch of OB-GYNs trying to fill the primary care gap points to a bigger problem with how the specialty itself is designed. OB-GYN sits in a space that no other field occupies.

It's considered a surgical field, but doesn't offer the extended training time most surgical disciplines require. It overlaps with primary care, but doesn't emphasize relationship building, chronic disease management, or behavioral health in the same way family medicine does. It touches mental health, sexual health, and identity—but rarely goes deep enough to offer comprehensive care in those areas.

And then there's the history. The specialty wasn't created out of patient need, it was cobbled together for institutional convenience. Instead of separating out breast health, gynecology, pregnancy, hormones, and menopause, medicine lumped them all under one umbrella and called it OB-GYN.

Think about what we're actually asking OB-GYNs to do. They're expected to be surgeons who can perform complex operations and emergency C-sections. They're expected to be primary care doctors who manage blood pressure and depression screening. They're expected to be fertility specialists who understand the latest reproductive technologies.

They're expected to be trauma-informed counselors who can navigate sexual assault histories and pregnancy loss. They're expected to be hormone experts who understand everything from adolescent development to menopause. They're expected to be labor managers who can handle high-risk deliveries and postpartum complications. The list goes on and on. The expectations are almost impossible.

When you step back and see the impossible scope of OB-GYN, and remember that the merger that created it was rooted more in institutional convenience than patient care, it's clear the gaps you feel in your appointments aren't personal. They're structural.

And you notice them in moments that matter: When chronic pelvic pain is dismissed as "normal," when postpartum anxiety is brushed off with "you just had a baby," when sexual side effects are met with silence. It's not that your provider doesn't care. It's that the system doesn't give them the training, the time, or the space to care in the ways you need.

## A Revealing Comparison: OB-GYN Versus Urology

To really understand how overstretched OB-GYN training is, it helps to compare it with another specialty that overlaps in both anatomy and procedure: urology.

Both OB-GYNs and urologists operate on the pelvic organs. Both manage hormone-related conditions, surgical interventions, fertility, pain, and sexual health. But if you look at what each specialty is actually expected to cover, and the differences become stark.

Urologists focus primarily on the genitourinary tract and related surgical conditions. Their scope is deep but relatively narrow: kidneys, bladder, urethra, and male reproductive organs. Most of their patients are adults with specific urologic problems.

OB-GYNs, by contrast, are expected to cover the entire reproductive life cycle for half the population, from adolescent development to menopause, and from fertility preservation to postpartum trauma recovery. They handle everything from routine Pap smears to emergency C-sections, from contraception counseling to cancer surgery.

And the training? Strikingly different.

Urology residencies typically last five to six years. They begin with one to two years of general surgery training, followed by four years of urology-specific training. That foundation provides a broad surgical education before narrowing into a specific focus on urologic systems.

Meanwhile OB-GYN trainees dive straight into specialty care from day one. They get just four years to cover the full spectrum of obstetrics and gynecology, without the added foundation of a surgical residency, and are expected to juggle it all: managing high-risk labor; performing complex operations; providing primary-care-level support for contraception, menopause, and mental health; and navigating both emergencies and chronic conditions.

A recent *JAMA Surgery* commentary went even further, arguing that gynecologic surgery should be its own residency. Right now, trainees split their time among deliveries, office visits, and the OR, often graduating without enough surgical volume to feel fully competent. When training is stretched this thin, it's patients who pay the price: with longer procedures, fewer minimally invasive options, and too few experts prepared to manage complex gynecologic disease.

## Looking Beyond Our Borders

Healthcare in the United States was never designed for true task sharing: a team-based model where midwives, advanced practice providers, family physicians, and specialists each practice to the top of their training, working together to share the load of care.

In many other countries, however, task sharing is the norm. Elsewhere, midwifery isn't treated as an alternative or a niche, it's a core part of the healthcare system. Midwives there are trained to handle low-risk pregnancies from start to finish, with obstetricians stepping in for complications or surgical needs.

That division of labor means OB-GYNs can focus more deeply on complex cases, while midwives build continuity and trust through longer visits and ongoing relationships. Patients get more time, more personalized attention, and a smoother handoff when higher-level care is needed.

Other systems lean more on family physicians with obstetric training to provide routine prenatal, postpartum, and gynecologic care, especially in rural or underserved areas. That creates a bridge between primary care and specialty care, something we often lose in the United States, where OB-GYNs and PCPs operate in silos.

Even within the United States, some hospitals and clinics are experimenting with more integrated models: OB-GYNs, midwives, nurse practitioners, family medicine physicians, and pelvic floor therapists working side by side, sharing records and patient goals. It's not perfect and it's far from the norm, but when it's done well, it enables each clinician to practice at the top of their license, rather than stretching one provider to do it all.

I was reminded of how different this looks abroad when a friend from physician associate (PA) school, who delivered her first baby in Texas, moved to the Netherlands and became pregnant with her second. The differences in her care are striking. In the Netherlands, routine pregnancy care is fully midwife-led and entirely covered by basic insurance. If complications arise or a prior C-section changes the risk profile, patients are referred to an OB in the hospital later in pregnancy.

Along the way, she received access to a dietitian and diabetic nurse when her glucose test was borderline, extra ultrasounds when growth needed monitoring, and a home health professional called a *kraamverzorgster*, part of the Dutch *kraamzorg* service, who comes daily for the first 8–10 days after birth. She helps with everything from baby care and breastfeeding to cooking and cleaning, so new parents can actually rest. It's tender, practical, and built into the very fabric of postpartum care. And all of it is fully covered by basic health insurance.

In the United States, by contrast, most new parents are sent home within days of delivery with a newborn in their arms, little support, and a six-week follow-up appointment circled on the calendar. As if recovery, feeding, and parenting can wait that long.

My friend's experience underscores how much infrastructure, philosophy, and training shape what care feels like. In these systems, preventive and low-risk care is built to be holistic, collaborative, and accessible, not an afterthought dependent on the bandwidth of a single OB-GYN.

Imagine if our system embraced that kind of collaboration on a national scale. OB-GYNs could train more deeply in high-risk pregnancy, complex surgery, fertility, and gynecologic disease. All without having to master every facet of preventive care, adolescent health, menopause, and sexual wellness in the same four-year residency. Advanced Practice Providers such as PAs, nurse practitioners, and midwives could handle more low-risk care, freeing up specialists for emergencies and complex cases. Family physicians could provide reproductive care alongside managing chronic conditions, making care more holistic and accessible.

But collaboration alone isn't the whole story, how we train providers shapes what follows, and the length and depth of OB-GYN training looks very different around the world. In the United States, medical school typically lasts four years, followed by four years of OB-GYN residency. Compare that to Ghana, where medical school is six years, followed by five years of residency. In the United Kingdom, medical school is usually five to six years, followed by seven years of specialty training in obstetrics and gynecology.

Aside from the curriculum and duration of training, rural care as a cornerstone of training is vastly absent in the United States. In Ghana, residents spend time in rural hospitals during their training, managing emergencies without the safety net of subspecialists or high-tech operating rooms. Turkey requires new graduates to work in rural areas for 300 to 500 days after training, meaning residents have to graduate ready to handle everything from complicated labor to ectopic pregnancy surgery on their own. In the United States, unless a resident chooses an elective away rotation, they may never train in a rural hospital at all, which is incredibly problematic as the United States is desperate for rural providers: over 35% of US counties are maternity care deserts with no obstetric coverage.

These task-sharing models, personal stories, and global training comparisons show us what's possible: a system in which care is better distributed, training is more comprehensive, and patients aren't left depending on a single overstretched specialist to do it all. But, alas, it's not what we have.

## The Limitations of the OB-GYN Residency

Residency is where the curriculum taught in medical school collides with the realities of the American healthcare system. It's where future OB-GYNs are asked to master everything from high-risk deliveries to complex pelvic surgeries, while also handling the bread-and-butter of routine reproductive care, all in just four years. The pace is relentless. Eighty-hour weeks aren't rare; they're often the expectation. Days start before sunrise, often end long after dark, and can be punctuated by middle-of-the-night calls that pull residents back into the hospital.

Residency isn't just intellectually demanding, it's emotionally punishing. Residents shoulder responsibility for two lives at once, and carrying the emotional weight of stillbirths, miscarriages, high-risk diagnoses, and traumatic deliveries. It requires sharp clinical instincts, surgical precision, and the ability to stay composed when everything is unraveling.

It's an environment that teaches stamina, precision, and quick decision-making. But it leaves little space for the slower, more relational parts of care. The parts of medicine that require you to sit down, listen, and connect. When the clock is always running, it's easier to focus on what's urgent than what may be important. And when the training window is short, the so-called optional topics like trauma-informed care, menopause, or nuanced conversations about sexual health get deprioritized.

Meanwhile, the scope of OB-GYN has exploded in the last two decades. Robotics. Advanced genetic counseling. Complex pregnancies involving heart disease or cancer. But while the to-do list keeps growing, training hours are shrinking. Hours are now capped at 80 per week in the United States, 48 in the European Union. Don't get me wrong, the training caps are necessary, the hourly toll is inhumane. But it means more to learn, less time to learn it, and a tendency toward knowing a little about everything, but deeply about less.

And here's the problem: when you're trying to fit obstetrics, gynecology, surgery, endocrinology, oncology, and emergency care into four years, and expecting residents to function on little sleep and nonstop pressure, there's simply not enough space left for the slower, relational parts of care. The parts that translate into you feeling seen and cared for. Because those are the very skills that shape patient experience.

The difference between healing and harm often comes down not just to what a provider does in the room, but how they enter it. And when training sidelines the human side of medicine, patients feel it. Every. Single. Day.

## When the System Decides What Fits and What Doesn't

I will pause here to acknowledge that I didn't go through OB-GYN residency myself. Those who did are the ones who know the real day-to-day sacrifices: the overnight calls, the relentless hours, and the weight of managing two lives at once. I have enormous respect for that, and for the fact that OB-GYNs emerge from that training as brilliant surgeons, diagnosticians, and advocates for their patients. What I'm describing here isn't a critique of their effort or commitment, it's about the structures that shape what's possible for them to learn.

And the data backs it up. National surveys of OB-GYN residents and program directors show that training is far from consistent. More than half of residents say they're dissatisfied with their education, and nearly 9 in 10 say it needs serious improvement. Program directors themselves agree: almost all believe every resident should have access to the same high-quality training, and most want a standardized national program to make that possible.

Even when programs try to do better, the system makes it nearly impossible to sustain. At one residency in Maine, faculty added a new project track where residents could design improvements for patient care. It worked. Human papillomavirus (HPV) vaccine counseling rates nearly doubled. But the only reason it survived was because a few faculty donated their time without extra support.

Another program tested an online module on high blood pressure in pregnancy. Residents scored higher on quizzes and ordered more labs, but they still weren't consistently counseling patients or prescribing needed medication. Without time, follow-up, or reinforcement, the gains faded. These are smart, committed doctors trying their best within limits most of us outside the system can't fully appreciate.

And the omissions aren't just in the "optional" topics. Ethics, a cornerstone of good care, barely gets covered. A national survey found most programs devoted fewer than five hours a year to it, often without structure. Nearly three-quarters of program directors wanted more ethics in residency, and 85% said it should be required. The barriers? Too little time, too few faculty, and a curriculum already bursting at the seams.

Menopause care tells the same story. Despite being a universal life stage, fewer than a third of OB-GYN programs had a menopause curriculum, and fewer than one in three offered residents time in a menopause clinic. More than 90% of program directors said standardized national training is needed. Again, this isn't about individual doctors deciding menopause doesn't matter, it's about how little space the system leaves for something so central.

The cracks start even earlier. A study of medical students preparing to enter OB-GYN found that fewer than one in four passed a standardized test of readiness. After a short elective course, most improved, but by the start of residency some of those gains had already slipped away, and not every school even offers such electives. That means new doctors are walking in with uneven preparation, through no fault of their own.

Even those who go on to fellowship for additional years of subspecialty training report that residency left them unevenly prepared. In a survey of nearly 500 fellows across maternal-fetal medicine, gynecologic oncology, reproductive endocrinology, and pelvic reconstructive surgery, about three-quarters said they felt prepared overall. But when asked about specific skills, gaps emerged. These are incredibly bright, dedicated physicians, but their training has holes not because they aren't capable, but because the structure doesn't cover everything.

And it's not just OB-GYN residencies. Many people rely on family physicians or internists for Pap smears, contraception, or pregnancy counseling. But a recent review of more than 100 studies found that women's health training in primary care residencies was just as fragmented: only a quarter of programs offered anything close to comprehensive training, most leaned heavily on lectures, and very few measured outcomes that mattered for patients.

The throughline is clear: what gets taught, and what doesn't, has little to do with patient need and everything to do with what the system makes possible. The silences you may have felt in your own appointments about menopause, trauma, miscarriage, or sexual health, are mirrored by silences in the syllabus. Not because doctors don't care, but because residency is built inside a scaffolding that ties their hands.

That scaffolding is made up of the rules and realities shaping every program: four years to cover an ever-expanding list of skills, hospital priorities that favor procedures over conversations, insurance systems that limit what care is modeled, laws and politics that erase entire areas of training overnight, and faculty already stretched too thin to add more. Put together, these structures decide what residents learn.

My goal here isn't to diminish OBGYNs themselves, but to highlight how these structural gaps ripple out into patient care. Until those structures shift, the gaps will remain, and patients will keep paying the price.

## The Pipeline Problem: Who Gets In, Who Stays, and Who Walks Away

Barriers exist in every level of training, shaping not only how many providers we have but also who those providers are. That matters, because when the people delivering care don't reflect the patients receiving it, trust erodes and outcomes suffer.

### Getting into Medical School

The first challenge begins with admission to medical school. Over a century ago, the Flexner Report of 1910 reshaped US medical education by changing academic requirements and mandating university training before medical school. It standardized the field and brought more scientific rigor, but it also shut the doors on many. Within a few years, more than half of all medical schools in the country closed. This included almost every school that had trained women, Black students, and lower-income students.

Medicine became a profession reserved for those with wealth and access, and that exclusivity still lingers. A century later, the pipeline remains skewed: in 2017, nearly half of US medical students came from families in the wealthiest 20% of the country, while students from the poorest 20% have never made up more than about 5% of a class.

For reproductive healthcare, the impact was profound. With women and people of color largely excluded from the profession, the specialty was shaped almost entirely through the lens of wealthy white men. Midwifery and community-based reproductive care were devalued, while surgical skill and pathology became the benchmarks of training. Those choices set a trajectory that still defines the field today: one where access is inequitable, diversity is limited, and relational, everyday reproductive care is often overshadowed by procedure-driven medicine.

Every step of the application process reflects income, privilege, and opportunity. The MCAT (a test required for admission to medical school) is expensive to prepare for, and scores correlate with family income. Research and shadowing opportunities disproportionately go to students with physician relatives or financial freedom to take on unpaid work. Even application fees, travel for interviews, and the costs of post-baccalaureate programs create additional hurdles. Meanwhile, one in five medical students has a parent who is a physician, connections that open doors unavailable to many first-generation or low-income students. The result is a pipeline where wealth and social capital shape who gets in, long before skill, compassion, or commitment to underserved communities can be measured.

## Getting into (and Through) OB-GYN Residency

Residency is where the pipeline narrows again, shutting out many of the candidates most needed in reproductive healthcare. OB-GYN residency slots are competitive. That might sound like a good thing since we want highly qualified people in these roles, but it has a hidden cost; the more competitive the match, the more the system favors candidates with built-in advantages: access to prestigious undergrad and medical schools, research opportunities, strong mentorship, and the financial freedom to bolster their résumé with unpaid electives, research, or externships.

That means people from underrepresented racial, socioeconomic, or geographic backgrounds, many of whom are most likely to return and serve the communities that need OB-GYNs most, continue to be systematically filtered out.

Furthermore, medical students may be drawn toward a higher-paying specialty, and it isn't hard to see why. Years of training come with staggering debt, often well into six figures, and many other specialties offer far higher salaries with fewer grueling hours than OB-GYN.

Payment structures make this problem worse. A *JAMA Surgery* analysis found that procedures performed on female patients are reimbursed up to 30% less than comparable surgeries on male patients. That gap doesn't just devalue women's health, it actively steers physicians away from gynecologic surgery as a specialty, deepening workforce shortages and leaving patients with fewer options for timely, high-quality care.

The trade-offs are clear: in OB-GYN, nights and weekends are rarely protected, malpractice premiums are higher, and the emotional toll of caring for patients through miscarriage, abortion, infertility, and maternal mortality can be crushing. Let alone now they have to practice in a polarizing political landscape. For students staring down decades of loan repayment, the financial calculations often push them elsewhere, even if they're passionate about reproductive health.

### *Working in Rural and Underserved Areas*

For those who do choose OB-GYN and survive residency, an additional barrier to having ample care across the United States is where providers end up practicing. New physicians can have debt that rivals a mortgage, which often nudges them toward urban centers rather than the rural counties where OB-GYNs are needed most. Loan forgiveness programs exist, but they're limited, inconsistent, and full of fine print that makes them hard to rely on.

For those who do choose underserved areas, burnout looms large. The emotional weight of reproductive healthcare is heavy everywhere, but in rural clinics or politically hostile states the load is crushing. Providers face overwhelming patient demand, fewer resources, longer hours, and in some places harassment or legal risk. Many leave after only a few years, creating a cycle where counties already struggling to recruit end up with no practicing OB-GYN at all. Patients are left driving hours just to receive routine prenatal care, and whole communities lose access to essential services.

So when we talk about "gaps" in the system, it's not just about what's missing in the curriculum. It's also about the bottleneck points in the pipeline: who gets trained, where they can afford to work, and how long they can survive in the job before the system grinds them down.

## Training Gaps in Reproductive Healthcare

The vast majority of OB-GYNs want to do right by their patients. They want to offer compassionate care. But they've been trained in a system that prioritizes diagnoses over dialogue, surgery over relationship building, and outcomes over emotional safety. They're taught to treat emergencies and save lives, but less emphasis is placed on prioritizing dignity in the process.

Some will argue that you can't expect medical school or residency to teach everything. Medicine is a lifelong education.

And that's true. Clinicians are always updating their knowledge as science evolves. But here's the catch: what gets prioritized in formal training shapes everything that comes after. If something is treated as foundational like surgical technique or managing high-risk pregnancy, physicians keep refining those skills throughout their careers. If something is treated as optional or skipped altogether, it almost never gets revisited.

A resident who was never trained to counsel a patient about sexual function or perimenopause isn't likely to seek it out later, because the system already told them it wasn't essential. The starting curriculum is like a compass. It sets the direction. And when that compass leaves out entire dimensions of care, most providers will never veer off course to find them.

This section looks at this issue through the lens of abortion training because that's where the gaps show up most starkly, but the same pattern applies across many other areas of reproductive healthcare. What's missing at the foundation rarely gets picked up later.

Organizations like Repro TLC work to provide the training that medical schools and hospitals so often neglect. In the case of Repro TLC, that means teaching how to provide abortion and miscarriage care safely, how to center a patient's voice in moments of crisis, how to practice trauma-informed care when bodies and lives are on the line. These aren't side skills or "nice to haves." They are the core realities of reproductive healthcare. Yet providers often only encounter them if they seek out supplemental training.

I know this firsthand. Several years ago, I began taking trainings through Repro TLC myself. Their programs shaped not only the way I practice but also the way I understand what truly counts as essential in reproductive healthcare. Through them, I became an abortion doula, trained in trauma-informed care, and learned what it means to build LGBTQ+ allyship directly into the clinic space.

Latona Giwa, the executive director of Repro TLC, shared with me how their organization also emphasizes supporting clinicians early in their careers, before the habits of a broken system can calcify. They understand that when you lay a foundation that centers dignity, compassion, and equity, you change the course of a provider's entire practice.

The overturning of *Roe v. Wade* has only made this worse. The Accreditation Council for Graduate Medical Education requires that all OB-GYN residency programs make abortion training available. But here's the catch: residents can opt out if they have religious or moral objections. On top of that, some institutions, especially Catholic-affiliated hospitals, prohibit abortion training altogether. Those programs often rely on "out-rotations" at external clinics, but in states with bans, those rotations have become extremely limited or impossible.

Abortion skills aren't only about elective procedures. They are the exact same skills used to treat miscarriages, manage ectopic pregnancies, and stop life-threatening bleeding. When those skills aren't taught or practiced, patient safety is compromised far beyond the abortion context.

That means whether you end up with a doctor who can manage an emergency may come down to nothing more than where they trained, what their system allowed them to learn, and how that provider personally feels about abortion care.

Even in states where abortion remains legal, many providers finish training without clear knowledge of the laws in their own state or without meaningful hands-on experience. Some programs, especially those based at religiously affiliated hospitals, don't offer any procedural training at all. In restricted states, the situation is even more dire. Residents often report a near-total loss of exposure. Some are forced to travel across state lines, arrange temporary housing, and pay out of pocket just to gain the most basic experience, if they can arrange it at all. That kind of patchwork training system isn't just unfair to learners; it's unsafe for patients.

Med Students for Choice (MSFC) was founded in 1993 as a response to the significant deficit of abortion education in their medical training. Their goal was to connect medical students, no matter where they trained, to abortion and family planning education. Even before the overturning of *Roe*, most schools weren't required to provide it, and many outsourced it as an away elective. After the *Dobbs* decision, the training became even more scarce, and the organization shifted its focus to reshaping the training landscape and ensuring access to the education that was rapidly disappearing.

Pamela Merritt, executive director of MSFC, explained to me that they are now organizing to expand core curricula and pushing to make abortion training mandatory for accreditation in the United States. "The reproductive present and future of millions of Americans is at stake," she said. "Access to modern science-based and patient-centered care in 20 states is at stake. All patients deserve excellent physicians, and that requires a top-notch comprehensive education. Physicians can't save the life of a pregnant person if they haven't been trained and performed procedures in emergency situations."

Behind every statistic on maternal morbidity are real people whose futures are altered: people who lose their fertility, their health, or even their ability to work and care for their families. Delays in care carry consequences, and being forced to cross multiple states to access a basic medical service is, as Merritt described, "an indefensible burden on women and families."

## The Data We Don't Have and Why That's a Problem

Let's talk about the research. Or rather, the shocking lack of it.

Because even if a provider makes it through school, seeks out continuing education, and genuinely wants to offer better care, they're still often trying to build care on missing pieces. Why? Because we have shockingly little data on many things that matter in reproductive healthcare.

Despite making up more than half the population, women's health receives only about 8% to 11% of National Institutes of Health research funding. The consequences ripple through every aspect of care: across medicine, women have historically been underrepresented in clinical trials, which means that we lack critical data on how common conditions, medications, and interventions affect them specifically. Dosages are wrong. Side effects go unrecognized. Symptoms are misinterpreted. And care gets compromised.

Nowhere is that more glaring than in pregnancy. Of all industry-sponsored clinical trials in the United States in 2013, just 1% were designed specifically for pregnant women, and 98% of drug and device trials excluded them entirely. As a result, 85% of medications prescribed during pregnancy have never been studied for safety or efficacy in pregnant populations. This is not because we know they're harmful, but because we simply don't know.

Here's the bind: pregnant people face two kinds of risk. There's the potential risk of being included in clinical trials, where the effects of a drug or device might not be fully understood. And then there's the risk of being excluded. Taking medications that were never studied in pregnancy, with no data on dosing, safety, or side effects. Either way, the danger isn't always the medicine itself but the lack of evidence.

Medications are prescribed every day without pregnancy-specific data, not because people aren't using them, but because no one is collecting the outcomes. That's not protection. That's neglect disguised as caution.

The intent was to protect pregnant people from risk. But the result? Uncertainty. Fear. Guesswork. When research is missing, clinicians are left with vague recommendations, contradictory advice, and disclaimers in lieu of answers. We're not offering better care, we're avoiding liability.

There *are* ethical ways to include pregnant people in research, and there have been for decades. What's missing isn't safety, it's the will to build an infrastructure that makes it possible.

Ethical research doesn't mean enrolling pregnant patients in high-risk drug trials without context. It means ensuring informed consent, transparent risk communication, and appropriate monitoring, including pregnant people in observational studies and post-marketing surveillance, creating pregnancy-specific trial arms for widely used medications, and treating patients not just as subjects but as partners in knowledge building.

We don't need to choose between safety and evidence. We need research frameworks that treat pregnancy not as a legal risk, but as a clinical reality worthy of investment, transparency, and trust. We need the funding to back it up. We deserve more than disclaimers. We deserve data. We deserve clarity. We deserve answers.

Pregnancy highlights one form of exclusion, but it doesn't end there. People with underlying conditions like polycystic ovary syndrome (PCOS), fibroids, endometriosis, or autoimmune disorders are routinely excluded from large trials in the name of "reducing variability." But that variability isn't noise, it's reality. When you cut out complexity, you cut out the very people who live with it.

And it's bigger than individual conditions. Whole communities are erased from the data entirely, treated as outliers instead of essential voices.

Racial and ethnic minorities especially Black, Indigenous, and Latina women, are completely underrepresented across nearly every category of health research. And the consequences can be deadly. For example, Black women are 40% more likely to die from breast cancer than white women, yet they're significantly underrepresented in breast cancer clinical trials. Hispanic women are less likely to be screened for cervical cancer, despite higher rates of HPV-related cervical disease. Indigenous women experience some of the highest maternal mortality rates in the United States, yet data on their reproductive health outcomes remains limited and fragmented.

Expanding research to include diverse populations and the full spectrum of conditions isn't just equitable, it's essential. Without it, we keep building a medical system that only works for some, while leaving the rest to fall through the gaps.

## The Cycle of Invisibility

Here's the trap we're stuck in: if something isn't taught, it never enters the clinical imagination. Providers can't recognize what they were never trained to see, so it doesn't get diagnosed as frequently as it should. Without ample and appropriate diagnoses, conditions don't rise to the top of research agendas. And if they're not researched, they're written off as unimportant, justifying their absence in both textbooks and training.

Research is the gatekeeper. Only the conditions prioritized for funding are studied, while others are left out entirely. That's especially true in women's health, where research is negligible to begin with, gynecological conditions routinely receive only a fraction of the attention and dollars devoted to other fields. The lack of data is then used as proof that these conditions don't matter. Or worse, don't exist. Patients' lived experience alone rarely drives ample examination and exploration, so the gaps widen. And with no research to draw from, there's little justification for teaching the next generation of providers about those conditions at all.

This cycle of invisibility, illustrated in Figure 2.1, goes around and around, a cycle that keeps entire areas of reproductive healthcare invisible. What isn't researched doesn't get taught. What isn't

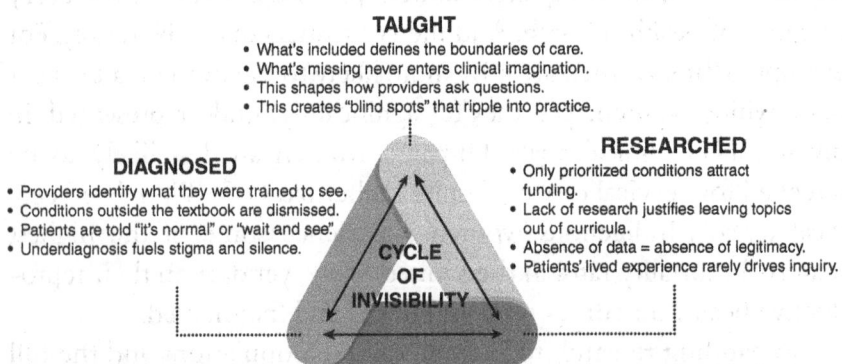

**Figure 2.1** The cycle of what is taught, diagnosed, and researched reinforces itself, erasing entire areas of reproductive healthcare from view.

taught doesn't get diagnosed. What isn't diagnosed doesn't get researched. A closed loop, self-reinforcing, shaping not just how providers are trained, but how patients are believed, diagnosed, treated, or ignored. Entire areas of reproductive healthcare disappear in this cycle, erased before they ever had a chance to be taken seriously.

## Case Study: Endometriosis and the Cost of Neglect

Endometriosis is one of the clearest examples of how the cycle of invisibility plays out in real time. An estimated 10% of people of reproductive age worldwide, roughly 190 million women and girls, may have endometriosis. And yet most will wait years, even decades, for recognition. That scale alone should make endometriosis a central focus in medicine. Instead, it's treated as an afterthought. Despite its prevalence, endometriosis is often dismissed as "just bad periods," ignored in research agendas, and overlooked in medical training.

What makes endometriosis such a powerful case study is not just its reach, but how clearly it exposes the cracks in the system: a condition this widespread should be impossible to miss, yet it routinely slips through the gaps of education, diagnosis, funding, and care.

**Taught:** Most medical students and residents receive only superficial instruction on endometriosis. Despite being a leading cause of pelvic pain and infertility worldwide, the disease is often reduced to a few slides in a single lecture.

**Diagnosed:** That lack of training translates directly into delay and harm. On average, patients wait 7–12 years and see three-plus clinicians before receiving a diagnosis. During those years, many are told their pain is just "bad periods," or worse, that it's all in their head. The delay isn't just frustrating; it robs people of fertility, intensifies chronic pain, and eliminates opportunities for earlier, more effective treatment.

**Researched:** Diagnosis gaps feed straight into funding gaps. Without enough cases formally recognized, conditions like endometriosis remain low on research agendas. "Endometriosis has historically received less research funding relative to its prevalence and impact than almost any other gynecologic condition." And in a field where women's health research is already minimal, falling behind here doesn't just slow progress, it pushes it even further out of view. Fewer diagnoses mean less data, less data leads to less funding, and less funding means fewer breakthroughs.

The consequences are devastating. Endometriosis doesn't just cause pain, it reshapes lives. It is one of the leading causes of pelvic pain and a major driver of infertility worldwide. Patients with endometriosis report higher rates of depression, anxiety, and relationship stress than their peers, and the disease is consistently tied to "marked decreases in quality of life, productivity, and increased healthcare utilization." This isn't just about cramps or difficult periods. It's about careers derailed, relationships strained, and families left in limbo. And yet, despite affecting millions, their suffering is still minimized.

Fixing this cycle requires more than sympathy, it demands systemic reform. Clinician education must move beyond a single lecture to include real training in diagnosis and management, with clear, evidence-based pathways that shorten the years-long delay patients face. Treatment should be coordinated through multidisciplinary models that bring together gynecology, pain management, mental health, gastroenterology, and fertility, so patients aren't left piecing care together on their own. And research priorities must finally reflect patient burden, with funding for noninvasive diagnostics, long-term outcomes, and better pain management. Treating endometriosis as a niche condition isn't just shortsighted, it's negligent.

## The Missing Pieces of Care

Endometriosis isn't the only example, it's just one piece of a much bigger pattern. I could build out that same model across nearly every corner of reproductive healthcare, because the gaps are everywhere: in training, in research, and inevitably in patient experience. When we start to pull those pieces apart, we see just how interwoven the neglect really is.

Take pelvic floor dysfunction: it affects nearly one in four women, yet it gets less than 2% of teaching time in urogynecology training. Or sexual pain disorders: they affect one in six, but fewer than a third of medical schools even teach students how to recognize or treat them. And those are only two examples out of dozens. Miscarriage, menopause, preeclampsia, perinatal mental health, chronic pelvic pain... the list goes on.

These aren't fringe issues. They're not niche. They're real, life-altering conditions patients bring into exam rooms every day. The tragedy isn't just that they've been left out, it's that their absence is used to justify continued neglect. We normalize the gaps, then blame patients for slipping through them.

Until we rewrite the loop, we'll keep failing the very people healthcare was meant to serve. And those failures won't just stay in textbooks or training modules. They'll show up in the real world: in missed diagnoses, rushed visits, pain that's brushed off, grief that's never acknowledged. They'll live in the stories patients carry long after the appointment ends.

What's missing in training becomes what's missing in care. And when you start to look, you'll see just how much has gone missing. We're going there next.

# Chapter 3

# Missing Pieces, Missing Care

*When Silence, Stigma, and Neglect Leave Patients "Unseen"*

We've already traced the dark history of reproductive healthcare, and we've seen how modern training continues to center procedures, speed, and technical mastery above all else. But when training is built this way, whole pillars of care get left out.

What remains can still hold up a roof, but the building itself has gaping holes. The structure may still stand, but with walls missing and patients left exposed. Care may be clinically correct yet incomplete, leaving questions half-answered, pain minimized, and lives outside the exam room ignored. What's missing isn't optional; it's the foundation that makes care human.

Whether we are talking about a universal stage of life like menopause or conditions that may not be fatal but can severely diminish your quality of life, including mental well-being, care is fragmented, underfunded, and left to chance. These gaps are not isolated oversights but part of a larger pattern: if an issue primarily affects women or marginalized communities, or doesn't fit neatly into a biomedical model, it's sidelined. That underinvestment doesn't just harm patients—it reverberates through families, workplaces, and the economy.

Investing in women's health changes the equation. Closing the gap could cut women's years in poor health by nearly two-thirds, boost the global economy by $1 trillion annually by 2040, and improve the lives of 3.9 billion women. Every dollar invested yields roughly three in return. This isn't a side issue; it's central to public health and economic stability.

That doesn't mean providers are unskilled or uncaring. It means their training is built for emergencies, not the everyday. They know how to stop hemorrhages, deliver babies, perform lifesaving surgeries. But many are far less prepared for the quieter, more human moments of care: supporting a patient miscarrying at home, talking through painful sex, or navigating the tender intersection of trauma and touch. These aren't failures of compassion—they're gaps in preparation. These are gaps that leave patients feeling unseen, and providers unaware of just how much they're missing.

And patients feel those gaps. In rushed visits, shrugged shoulders, unanswered questions. In pain dismissed, identities misunderstood, grief minimized.

This chapter looks at those missing pillars. The essential elements of reproductive care overlooked in training and, as a result, in practice. Once you see the blind spots, you can't unsee them. And once you know how much has been left out, it's clear why so many patients walk away unseen.

## Nonprioritized Yet Life-Changing Conditions

Some of the most common conditions in reproductive health cause massive disruption to daily life, and yet the system still treats them like side issues. If a diagnosis isn't considered "urgent" or "life-threatening" in a biomedical sense, it's brushed aside. The result? People lose years, sometimes decades, struggling with pain, bleeding, fatigue, or hormonal symptoms that could be treated or better managed if only they were taken seriously from the very beginning.

Patients leave their visits frustrated and unheard, disappointed that what's making it hard to work, parent, or even get out of bed wasn't considered "serious enough." The burden then falls back on them, forcing patients to repeatedly advocate for themselves while trying not to be dismissed as "difficult" or "needy." It's an exhausting cycle that leaves too many people questioning their own reality.

This dismissal has been ingrained in medical culture for decades. Doctors have shared stories of preceptors and advisors who had warned of the "whiny woman." WW became a shorthand used to write off patients who show up with multiple, overlapping symptoms like chronic pain, irregular bleeding, fatigue, brain fog, or sleep changes. Rather than recognizing these as red flags for conditions like endometriosis, polycystic ovary syndrome (PCOS), fibroids, perimenopause, or prolapse, providers too often attribute them to stress, mood, or simply getting older. The WW framing has left countless patients gaslit, untreated, and living with preventable suffering.

The truth is, these so-called side issues are not side issues at all, and sharing concerns about your quality of life is not whining. These conditions shape daily living in profound ways, influencing everything from fertility to mental health to economic stability. In the sections ahead, I'll unpack some of them—how they show up, why they've been ignored, and what it means for patients to finally have their experiences validated and addressed.

### *Menopause: The Unacknowledged Universal Experience*

Menopause is one of the only universal experiences for cisgender women, yet medical education continues to treat it like an elective topic. Despite the fact that every woman who lives long enough will go through it, menopause remains one of the most under-taught, under-researched, and misunderstood areas in reproductive health.

We treat puberty as a predictable transition. We give young people education, support, and a plan. We should do the same for menopause. Because this isn't a niche experience, it's inevitable. And it's time our medical system treated it that way.

Yet, less than a third of OB-GYN residency programs in the United States have a formal menopause curriculum. Let that sink in. The majority of doctors who specialize in women's reproductive health are never actually taught how to care for patients through menopause. The stage of life that affects half the population and can stretch on for decades.

Point blank: menopause is miserable for most. We've known that for a long time. We've studied it, documented how poorly it's treated, and yet the system has barely moved. In 2013, only about 20% of OB-GYN programs had a formal menopause curriculum. Ten years later, we've crawled up just 10 percentage points. That's it. At this pace, it will take 70 more years before every program training "women's health specialists" actually teaches them how to care for women in menopause. And that's if we even manage to keep making progress in today's political landscape.

Most women in the United States will go through menopause without ever seeing a provider truly trained to help. A majority of OB-GYNs say they feel ill-equipped to prescribe hormone therapy, and nearly three-quarters admit they're unsure how to manage complex menopausal symptoms. That leaves patients stuck in limbo, living with hot flashes, night sweats, and brain fog they assume are inevitable, or worse, fearing something more serious because no one gave them clear answers.

And this isn't just about today's doctors, it's about the pipeline. In one study, less than 7% of residents across OB-GYN, internal medicine, and family medicine felt adequately prepared to manage menopause. Think about that: we are sending doctors into practice, doctors who will collectively treat millions of women in menopause, with almost no preparation at all.

It means women drag themselves into doctor's offices with insomnia, brain fog that tanks their performance at work, and joint pain that makes even daily tasks exhausting, only to be told they're stressed, anxious, or just "getting older." It means that when they ask about hormone therapy, their provider might hesitate, change the subject, or steer them away based on outdated fears or incorrect guidelines instead of current evidence. It means early menopause after hysterectomy or chemotherapy often goes unrecognized. It means vaginal dryness, painful sex, and urinary changes go untreated, not because they're unsolvable, but because no one ever taught the doctor how to bring them up or treat them.

And let's not forget that menopause isn't just about "old age." Perimenopause, the transition into menopause, often begins in the late 30s or early 40s and can stretch on for a decade or more. The average age of menopause is 51, but for some women it comes earlier, whether naturally or because of surgery, cancer treatments, or certain health conditions. That means women can spend nearly half their adult lives in the hormonal shifts of perimenopause, menopause, and postmenopause combined.

The current system is failing peri- and menopausal women. These are years marked by major hormonal shifts that affect everything from sleep and mood to metabolism, bone health, and cardiovascular risk. Yet instead of being met with thoughtful, evidence-based care, too many women are brushed off, told their symptoms are "just aging," or handed a one-size-fits-all solution that doesn't actually address their needs. The lack of training, research, and clinical attention leaves patients navigating hot flashes, brain fog, joint pain, and sexual health concerns largely on their own—forced to piece together answers from friends, social media, or trial and error. In this section, we'll explore how medicine's blind spots about menopause translate into real-world harm, and what's at stake when an entire stage of life is neglected by the healthcare system.

### Hormone Therapy: Lost in Misinformation

Hormone therapy (HRT) is one of the clearest examples of what gets lost when menopause care is treated as optional. For many women, it can be life-changing: relieving hot flashes, easing night sweats, improving sleep, protecting bone health, and helping with vaginal dryness and painful sex. And yet most women are never offered it as a real option. Too often, the conversation ends before it even begins.

That silence didn't happen by accident. It traces back to the 2002 Women's Health Initiative (WHI), which concluded that hormone therapy increased risks of breast cancer, stroke, and heart disease. What those headlines left out was context: the study enrolled women in their mid-60s, long past the natural menopausal transition, and relied on older, higher-dose oral formulations that are rarely used today. Even so, the findings triggered a seismic shift. Prescriptions dropped overnight, and the FDA added a black box warning—the strongest level of caution—to every estrogen product, including low-dose vaginal estrogen that barely enters the bloodstream.

A full generation of clinicians trained under that cloud of fear. For many, the safest option became avoidance. Meanwhile, research kept moving. Over two decades, a more nuanced picture emerged. One in which the timing of therapy, the kind of hormones used, and how they're delivered all shape risk. Starting systemic therapy closer to menopause appears safer for the heart than starting years later. Transdermal estradiol and micronized progesterone, which are more commonly prescribed today, likely carry lower cardiovascular and clotting risks than the older synthetic regimens used in the WHI. And vaginal estrogen has minimal systemic absorption at any age, including for women in their seventies and eighties.

In 2025, the FDA removed the black box warning. An acknowledgment that the old, blanket message about risk was outdated. It doesn't mean hormone therapy is risk-free or that it's right for everyone. It means the science is more complex than the warning label allowed. But a label change cannot fix what's still missing: most clinicians were never trained to talk about menopause in the first place. Many still feel uncertain, uncomfortable, or out-of date. Patients are left to search for answers alone, scrolling through social media, comparing notes with friends, or piecing together contradictory advice online.

The cost of that silence is enormous. Three-quarters of women say menopause has forced real changes in their daily lives, and more than half say it negatively affects them at work. Nearly 1 in 10 midlife women has taken time off because of unmanaged symptoms, contributing to billions in lost productivity every year. Women in their peak working and caregiving years are stepping back, not because they lack ambition, but because the system has failed to support them through a universal transition.

Hormone therapy isn't right for everyone, and it shouldn't be presented as a miracle fix. But women deserve honest, evidence-based conversations about risks and benefits, not avoidance rooted in decades-old fear. The removal of the black box warning is a step toward restoring access, but the real shift will come only when clinicians are trained to understand menopause, patients feel empowered to ask questions, and we finally treat this stage of life as a core part of healthcare, not an afterthought.

### *Inequities Within the Menopause Experience*

The disparities in menopause are even sharper for women of color. Studies show that Black women experience more frequent and intense hot flashes, night sweats, and sleep disruption, along with higher rates of depression, anxiety, and complications from chronic conditions like pain, diabetes, and cardiovascular disease.

Yet despite this evidence, their experiences remain underrepresented in research and underemphasized in medical training. Layer on the weight of structural inequities, socioeconomic barriers, and long-held stereotypes about menopause that disproportionately harm Black women and other marginalized groups, and the result is predictable: a life stage that is harder to navigate and far less likely to receive adequate care.

## *Fibroids and Endometriosis*

Fibroids and endometriosis are two of the most common reasons people end up in a gynecologist's office. Fibroids alone will affect the majority of women in their lifetime: more than 70% of white women and 84% of Black women by age 50. Black women are also more likely to develop them at a younger age, with larger and more numerous benign tumors, and are more likely to need surgery as treatment. Endometriosis affects at least 1 in 10 reproductive-age women, and likely more, given how often it goes undiagnosed for years.

Both conditions can cause heavy bleeding, bloating, anemia, infertility, and a long list of day-to-day disruptions. Endometriosis, in particular, is notorious for causing debilitating pain. Yet because neither condition is cancer, they often get pushed down the priority list. "Benign" in the chart too often translates into "you can live with it" in real life.

And so the recommendation is usually the same: try birth control, wait, see what happens. Surgery, whether myomectomy, hysterectomy, or excision, is treated as a last resort, even if it's clearly needed. In her book *Get It Out*, sociologist Andrea Becker highlights the jarring statistic that 90% of hysterectomies are classified as "elective." That label makes it sound like a convenience or a luxury, something optional, rather than what it often is: the only treatment that could finally stop debilitating pain and bleeding.

For people with conditions like fibroids or endometriosis, a hysterectomy isn't elective at all; it's lifesaving. The "elective" label has nothing to do with patient choice. It's about insurance coding, reimbursement, and a medical culture that still doesn't treat gynecologic suffering as urgent enough.

It's true that surgery isn't always the answer, and it's a good thing we have less invasive options to try first. But those options shouldn't be used as a reason to gatekeep surgery or to gaslight people into thinking their symptoms aren't "bad enough" yet. The problem isn't whether surgery comes first or last, it's that patients so often feel excluded from the decision-making altogether.

Add to that the fact that many general gynecologists aren't trained in advanced surgical techniques for endometriosis, and you've got a recipe for continued delay and dismissal. People are forced to go from one doctor to another, collecting half-answers and temporary fixes until they finally land in the right office. All the while, they've had to plan their lives around their symptoms and suffering.

"Benign" doesn't mean harmless. And until we start acting like that's true, patients will keep losing years to pain they didn't have to live with.

### *Perinatal Mental Health: A Silent Crisis*

Perinatal mental health isn't a side note, it's become the number one complication of childbearing. And yet in the United States, it's treated like an afterthought. Nearly one in five women will experience depression or anxiety during pregnancy or the year after giving birth. That's three to four times more common than either gestational diabetes (5–8%) or preeclampsia (5–7%), both of which we routinely screen for. But perinatal depression? Screening is patchy at best, and treatment often nonexistent.

All because the medical system keeps looking the other way. Most OB-GYNs aren't trained to spot these issues in the first place. Fewer than one in five residency directors believe their residents get adequate training in perinatal mental health. And when providers aren't prepared, patients fall through the cracks. More than half of perinatal mental health conditions go undiagnosed. That translates to as many as 600,000 new parents every single year struggling with untreated depression or anxiety while trying to care for a newborn.

This gap is deadly. Suicide is now a leading cause of maternal death in the United States, and perinatal mental health disorders are consistently called the most common complication of childbearing. It is unacceptable. And it is entirely preventable. We know how to screen. We know how to treat. We know that timely interventions save lives, protect children, and strengthen families. The only reason suicide remains a leading cause of maternal death is because of collective neglect. A healthcare system that has decided, over and over again, that mothers' mental health isn't the priority.

And the neglect lands hardest on the people who need help the most. Nearly half of all births in the United States are covered by Medicaid, yet only three states cover proven supports like doulas or community health workers, despite overwhelming evidence that these interventions save lives and reduce costs. In most states, coverage cuts off just 60 days postpartum, right when the risk of postpartum depression is at its highest. The result is a rigged, two-tier system: families with resources can buy help, while the most vulnerable mothers, the ones at highest risk, are left without.

Here's how this plays out in real life: a first-time mom shows up to her six-week postpartum check, the only appointment that's really for her after giving birth. The last time anyone asked about her mental health was a single screening form, rushed through before she was discharged from the hospital 24 hours after delivery. That was before the sleepless nights. Before the breastfeeding struggles. Before the financial stress of unpaid leave.

Now she hasn't slept more than two hours at a time in weeks. Her mind races at night, her chest feels heavy with dread, and sometimes she wonders if her baby would be better off without her. But the visit isn't about that. The conversation is about stitches, bleeding, contraception. Maybe a quick glance at the baby. No one asks how she's really doing. The doctor tells her she's "cleared" for sex. She forces a smile, nods politely. Inside, she's thought about hurting herself 20 times and not once about sex.

She gathers her diaper bag and heads for the parking lot. Minutes later, she's sobbing in her car. Alone. Exhausted. Already rehearsing how to hide her pain when she walks through the door. If you're a mother you know that this really isn't that hard to imagine.

Now imagine she's on Medicaid. Four weeks later, she's finally ready to say it out loud: she's not okay, she needs help. She calls her OB-GYN's office, only to be told her coverage ended two weeks ago. No visit. No care. The message is clear: her pain, her fear, her safety no longer matter.

Maybe this is your sister. Maybe it's your daughter. Maybe it was you, and you didn't recognize it at the time. That's what happens when a system decides mothers' mental health is disposable, and unfortunately it's far too easy to see how it plays out.

## *Beyond Childbearing: Mental Health Across the Reproductive Lifespan*

Perinatal mental health is only one piece of a much larger puzzle. The truth is, mental health challenges thread through nearly every phase of reproductive life, but they rarely get the attention they deserve.

Take fertility challenges and pregnancy loss. The grief of month after month of failed treatments, or the devastation of a miscarriage, doesn't just live in the body, it lives in the mind. Depression and anxiety rates spike, yet mental healthcare is often missing from fertility clinics or miscarriage management. Patients are left carrying invisible losses, sometimes with the added weight of silence and shame.

Premenstrual syndrome (PMS) and its more severe counterpart, premenstrual dysphoric disorder (PMDD), are another example of how symptoms are written off as "just hormones" or "just moodiness." For some, PMS is a mild inconvenience; for others, PMDD brings debilitating depression, rage, or despair that recurs every single month. Despite affecting up to 5–8% of menstruating women, PMDD remains underdiagnosed and undertreated, leaving patients to navigate cycles of suffering without real support.

Perimenopause and menopause bring their own terrain of risk. Mood swings, sleep disruption, and brain fog aren't just nuisances, they can be precursors to anxiety and depression. Add in the cultural stigma that frames menopause as decline, and women are left with little validation that what they're experiencing is both real and treatable. The lack of provider training here means too many midlife women are dismissed instead of supported.

Chronic reproductive conditions like endometriosis, PCOS, and fibroids also carry a heavy mental health toll. Living with pain, irregular bleeding, infertility, or repeated dismissal by the medical system chips away at resilience over time. The psychological burden isn't just secondary, it's part of the disease itself, even if medicine refuses to see it that way.

And layered across all of this are the mental health impacts of abortion bans. Being forced to continue a pregnancy against your will, or being denied care in the middle of a miscarriage, is traumatic. Research consistently shows that people denied abortions have worse mental health outcomes than those who receive them, and yet policy decisions are being made as if the psychological stakes don't matter.

Mental health doesn't exist in isolation from reproductive health, it's woven into every stage. Recognizing this isn't optional; it's the only way to build a system that actually cares for the whole patient, across their whole life.

### *Sexual Health: The Missing Conversation*

Sexual health education in medical training stays in a narrow lane: sexually transmitted infections (STIs), birth control methods, fertility. The rest—pleasure, desire, arousal, orgasm, intimacy—is either ignored or treated as irrelevant. A national survey of OB-GYN residency program directors found that fewer than half offered any formal curriculum on female sexual function, and most cited lack of training among faculty as the biggest barrier. In other words, the very people teaching tomorrow's doctors don't feel prepared to talk about sexual health themselves.

The result is a profession that can screen for chlamydia but stumbles when a patient brings up painful sex, low libido, or changes in arousal. Too often, women are brushed off with quick fixes. They're told "try lube," "it's probably hormonal," instead of receiving thoughtful, evidence-based care.

Sexual well-being is not optional. It's directly tied to mental health, physical health, and overall quality of life. When the medical system and the school system both reduce sexual health to nothing more than pregnancy prevention or infection control, they leave a void that women feel in their bodies, their relationships, and their sense of self every single day. What gets missed is everything beneath the surface: relationship dynamics, medication side effects, trauma history, vaginal atrophy, pelvic floor dysfunction.

And it's not just medical training that falls silent. It's a cultural gap. One that starts much earlier, in how we're taught about our own bodies. Most women grow up with little real education about sexual health beyond pregnancy and STIs. For decades, classrooms featured *The Miracle of Life* as the cornerstone of sex ed, a graphic birthing video paired with abstinence-heavy, fear-mongering lessons about sexually transmitted infections. The message was clear: sex was about risks and reproduction, not connection or pleasure. By the time many women enter the exam room, most don't even have the language to describe their concerns, let alone the confidence to ask for help.

It doesn't have to be this way. In the Netherlands, sex education starts in preschool and builds in an age-appropriate way. Early lessons focus on consent, boundaries, and what feels comfortable or uncomfortable, even something as simple as a friend sitting too close. An expat I spoke to shared that they don't just teach kids how to say no, they also teach them how to say yes. They teach them to understand and affirm what feels good, safe, and right. That shift in framing matters. Dutch teens grow up with the tools to talk about sex as something rooted in agency and connection, and the country has one of the lowest teenage pregnancy rates in the world to show for it.

The fallout of this silence in the United States is staggering. When sex ed skips over pleasure and intimacy, and when doctors are never trained to ask about them either, women carry that gap straight into adulthood. A nationally representative survey of more than 31,000 US women found that 43% reported at least one sexual problem, low desire, difficulty with arousal, pain with sex, or trouble reaching orgasm, yet only 22% reported distress about those problems. These aren't rare complaints; they're everyday realities that most women will face at some point, yet most have never been given the language, tools, or support to address them.

Behind those numbers are real lives: women avoiding intimacy because it hurts, partners feeling distant, parents juggling exhaustion and brain fog while quietly wondering if something is broken in them or if their relationship is failing. Instead of validation or treatment, they're too often dismissed with quick fixes. They're told "it's just hormonal," "it's normal for your age."

The truth is, sexual health is complex. And it is deeply connected to both physical and emotional well-being. But most providers were never trained to see it that way or to even begin the conversation, especially with women. That is not a minor oversight. It is a moral failure. It is a societal failure. And it is a curriculum failure.

But most of all, it's a failure you should never have to internalize. If you've struggled with desire, with pain, with intimacy that feels harder than it should—you are not broken. You are not "just hormonal." You are not alone. The silence about sexual health has left too many women carrying shame that was never theirs to carry.

Here's where the double standard comes into sharp focus. When men struggle with sexual function, the system springs into action. Erectile dysfunction was declared a public health priority, unlocking billions in research and a dozen FDA-approved medications—cheap, accessible, and covered by insurance. The message couldn't be clearer: men's sexuality is urgent, biomedical, and fixable.

But when women bring up the same concerns of desire, arousal, orgasm, and pain they're met with shrugs, stigma, or silence. Flibanserin/Addyi, the so-called female Viagra, took nearly two decades and relentless advocacy just to crawl across the finish line, despite showing comparable efficacy to drugs for men. And even now, treatments for women's sexual dysfunction remain scarce, expensive, and rarely covered. The difference cuts deeper than coverage. It says men's pleasure is a priority and women's is negotiable. Men's sexuality is treated like a right. Women's is treated like an afterthought.

The takeaway isn't just that the system has failed women, it's that women have refused to accept that failure. Addyi exists only because women demanded it. The fact that sexual health is even on the table in medicine today is because patients, advocates, and providers refused to shut up or back down. Men's pleasure has been treated like a birthright. Women's pleasure has been treated like a bargaining chip. It's not. Women's sexuality is not optional, not secondary, not negotiable. It's a right.

### *Prevention of High-Risk STIs*

You deserve care that treats sexual health as health. Not as a luxury, not as an indulgence, not as an afterthought, and certainly not as a point of shame for enjoying a sex life in the first place. Your pleasure, your desire, your comfort in your own body are essential parts of your well-being. Your body deserves joy, your relationships deserve intimacy, and you deserve to feel fully at home in yourself, which means having the right to protect it. But too often, the very tools that safeguard women's health are hidden behind stigma and silence.

And here's where silence shows up: the human papillomavirus (HPV) vaccine. HPV is one of the most common sexually transmitted infections, so common that before vaccination, nearly everyone was expected to be infected at some point in their lives. Most infections clear on their own, but persistent high-risk HPV types can cause several cancers, including cervical, vulvar, vaginal, anal, and oral cancers. In fact, HPV is linked to over 90% of cervical cancers.

The first HPV vaccine, Gardasil, was approved in 2006 for girls and young women up to age 26, and later expanded to include boys and adults up to age 45. The current version, Gardasil 9, is more than 90% effective at preventing infection by the nine HPV types most likely to cause cancer.

So why are so many women in their 30s and 40s still not being offered the vaccine? Because providers make assumptions. They assume a divorced or widowed patient isn't dating again. They dodge the conversation because it feels uncomfortable. And heaven forbid they consider that a woman over 40 might have new partners or be in an open or polyamorous relationship. That silence isn't neutral, it's stigma. Multiple partners are still coded as "promiscuous" instead of recognized as a normal reality for many adults, including those in committed, ethical, non-monogamous relationships. When providers won't talk about it, prevention never even makes it onto the table. Add in inconsistent insurance coverage after age 26, where the vaccine can cost hundreds of dollars per dose out of pocket, and women are left paying the price, in dollars and in health, for a system that still polices their sexuality.

The same silence shows up with HIV prevention. PrEP, an incredibly effective daily pill that reduces the risk of HIV by more than 90%, is rarely offered to women. It's not that women don't qualify; it's that providers don't often bring it up. They're far more likely to recommend PrEP to men who have sex with men than to women with male partners, even though women remain at risk. Once again, women's sexuality is treated as an afterthought, something too uncomfortable for providers to talk about, even when the stakes are life or death.

And HPV and HIV aren't the only infections in which silence costs women dearly. Chlamydia and gonorrhea can be silent for years but can cause pelvic inflammatory disease and infertility if left untreated. Herpes carries not only the burden of recurrent outbreaks but also the stigma that isolates patients and silences conversations. These infections are common, they are treatable, and in many cases preventable. But only if women are given accurate information and proactive care.

When prevention, testing, and treatment are treated as taboo, women pay the price in missed opportunities, chronic illness, and unnecessary suffering.

### *Substance Use: Stigma and Silence in the Exam Room*

Substance use is part of the reproductive health landscape, but you wouldn't know it from most OB-GYN visits. Conversations about alcohol, cannabis, prescription medications, or other drugs are either rushed, judgmental, or avoided altogether. Patients who try to bring it up often hear blanket discouragement instead of real counseling, by which I mean nonjudgmental screening, harm-reduction strategies, safety planning, and referrals to treatment when needed. When silence takes the place of honest dialogue, patients stop disclosing, and opportunities to protect health are lost.

Take marijuana. More and more states have legalized recreational use, yet most OB-GYN conversations haven't caught up. Patients who disclose cannabis use, whether for sleep, anxiety, pain, or recreation, are still often met with judgment, vague warnings, or silence. Instead of acknowledging legal status, frequency of use, and individual health needs, providers fall back on discomfort or stigma. Real counseling here should mean talking through potential risks in pregnancy or while breastfeeding, safer alternatives if available, and support for patients who want to cut back or quit. But when that doesn't happen, many patients just don't bring it up at all.

That same stigma extends to other forms of substance use, especially during pregnancy. While pregnancy is often described as a critical window to support people with substance use disorders, care rarely meets that moment with compassion or competence. Instead, many patients fear being reported, criminalized, or losing custody. So they either avoid care or stay silent with their clinicians.

In a 2019 qualitative study at Johns Hopkins, pregnant women with substance use disorders said they were motivated to seek treatment by concern for their baby's health, desire to regain custody, access to shelter or structure, and readiness to stop using. But the barriers were just as clear: stigma, fear of judgment, lack of childcare or transportation, and the very real risk of Child Protective Services involvement.

Despite growing evidence that comprehensive treatment improves outcomes for both parent and baby, most OB-GYNs receive little training in substance use: how to screen nonjudgmentally, how to provide harm-reduction counseling, how to connect patients to medication-assisted treatment like methadone or buprenorphine, or how to integrate care with behavioral health and social supports. This silence, whether concerning marijuana, methadone, or other substances, leaves patients isolated, afraid, and less likely to seek care when they need it most. Breaking that silence isn't optional; it's essential to ensuring safe, compassionate, and effective care for women and their families.

### *Hidden Abuse: What Clinicians Often Miss*

Abuse doesn't always show up as bruises or broken bones. In reproductive healthcare, it often hides in the choices patients aren't allowed to make or the ways their bodies are controlled by someone else. Yet medical training rarely teaches clinicians to see these hidden forms, much less how to respond to them.

Reproductive coercion is when a partner tries to control someone else's reproductive choices. Things like pressuring them not to use birth control, tampering with contraception, or forcing decisions about pregnancy outcomes. A study of women ages 18 to 44 in a large urban OB-GYN clinic found that about 16% reported experiencing reproductive coercion at some point in their lives.

Among those, nearly one in three (32%) also experienced intimate partner violence in the same relationship.

Despite those numbers, most OB-GYNs are never trained to screen for it, and many have never even heard the term. Without that language or awareness, what should be recognized as abuse often gets missed entirely.

Or consider trafficking. Research shows that the vast majority of trafficking survivors, about 90%, access medical care at some point while they're still being exploited. That means providers are seeing these patients regularly, sometimes in OB-GYN clinics, and not realizing what's happening. A lack of training on trafficking, combined with rushed visits and discomfort about asking sensitive questions, creates a blind spot exactly where vigilance is most needed.

The consequences are profound. When reproductive coercion and trafficking go unrecognized, patients don't just lose autonomy, they lose safety, health, and in some cases, their lives. And providers lose the chance to intervene at the very moments when their presence could matter most.

Yet the gap in training persists. Screening protocols, counseling strategies, and trauma-informed approaches are rarely standardized. If they're taught at all. As a result, clinicians enter exam rooms fully prepared to save lives in a medical emergency, but not to recognize when a patient's choices about sex, contraception, or pregnancy are being restricted or manipulated by someone else. That, too, is a crisis, just a different kind.

## When Pain Is Minimized, Not Managed

Pain is one of the most common reasons people seek reproductive healthcare, and one of the least addressed. Research shows that patients frequently experience moderate to severe pain during gynecologic procedures, with endometrial biopsies showing pain scores of 5–7 on a 10-point scale, and nearly 80% of women reporting moderate to severe pain during in intrauterine device (IUD) insertion if they've never given birth. Colposcopies, performed after an abnormal Pap smear, are often described as "minor" procedures, yet many patients report sharp, burning pain that lingers for days, with little preparation or relief offered in advance.

And it doesn't stop in the procedure room. Too often, patients are sent home from reproductive procedures with little more than ibuprofen, whether after an egg retrieval, a dilation and curettage (D&C), or even a C-section. Across the board, pain is minimized, undertreated, and dismissed. This leaves patients to manage not only their recovery, but the message that their suffering is somehow expected or acceptable.

And for Black patients, it's worse. Decades of research show they are less likely to have their pain taken seriously, less likely to receive adequate medication, and more likely to be dismissed when they speak up. Even after C-sections, the most common surgical procedure in the United States, Black women are discharged with fewer pain medications than white women, despite having undergone the exact same surgery. What is brushed off as "normal" discomfort for everyone becomes, for Black patients, a dangerous combination of neglect and bias that compounds the risks they already face in maternal health.

This reality was brought into national focus through the award-winning podcast *The Retrievals*. In its first season, host Susan Burton uncovered a chilling story: dozens of women undergoing fertility treatment at Yale reported feeling excruciating pain during egg retrievals, only to learn they had been given saline instead of fentanyl by a nurse who was stealing the medication for herself. But what resonated most was how quickly their reports of "something being wrong" were brushed aside. After the podcast aired, hundreds of listeners wrote in to share their own stories, some even describing the unthinkable: feeling every cut and tug during their C-sections.

The podcast laid bare what many patients already knew: women's pain is often normalized as "just part of the process" or outright ignored. It proved that this wasn't just a Yale story, it was a cultural one. Listeners across generations wrote in about IUD insertions, birth trauma, and everyday procedures where their pain was minimized, showing that the problem is systemic, not exceptional.

From period cramps to IUD placements, from endometriosis flares to post-op healing, patients are often told to expect pain instead of being offered relief. Too often, the language itself minimizes what's ahead. Providers say "you'll feel some pressure" when what many feel is sharp, burning pain. That gap between words and reality leaves patients blindsided, questioning their own reactions. And when they do speak up? They're often told it's normal. Or in their head. Or just something to get through. Providers default to reassurance, heating pads, or over-the-counter meds. Providers rarely offer more comprehensive options.

This isn't rare, it's systemic. A 2024 survey published in *BMJ Open* found that 77% of women reported having their pain dismissed or minimized by healthcare professionals at some point in their lives. That staggering number makes it clear: pain is still treated as subjective, unreliable, or exaggerated. Something to tolerate, not something to treat. This dismissiveness delays diagnoses, undermines treatment, and leaves lasting scars on both health and trust.

And it's not just medicine, it's culture. Women's pain, especially menstrual and gynecologic pain, is framed as "just a period," "just hormones," or "just part of being a woman." That language doesn't just minimize pain, it erases it. It conditions patients to accept suffering as normal, and conditions providers to overlook it before the exam even begins.

Until 2025, there were no national guidelines in the United States specifically addressing pain management for routine OB-GYN procedures. The fact that it took this long says everything: women's pain hasn't been prioritized or taken seriously for far too long. That delay hasn't just caused physical discomfort, it has eroded trust in the entire system.

And here's the double standard. When my husband needed a vasectomy, a quick, outpatient procedure, he was offered full anesthesia. It was done in a surgery center, billed through insurance, wrapped in comfort, even though many men describe the procedure as relatively simple. I'm glad he had a good experience, he gets queasy with a blood draw, so that level of care made sense for him. But that same benefit, that same presumption of comfort, should be extended to women, too.

The message is clear: men's pain is something to prevent. Women's pain is something to endure. That isn't medicine. That's bias. Plain and simple.

## The "Big Picture" That Medicine Still Misses

True comprehensive healthcare requires seeing the whole person, not just their symptoms. But that shift in mindset, from "What's wrong with your body?" to "How does your whole life shape your health?", is still missing in most exam rooms. And when providers don't zoom out, the stakes are high: care plans collapse in real life.

Picture this: a patient comes in with painful, heavy periods. Her provider rushes out the door and hands her a prescription for birth control pills. What never gets asked? That she's working two jobs without insurance, making the prescription unaffordable. That she has migraines, which the pill has worsened before. That she's been thinking about trying to get pregnant. In theory, the plan makes sense. In practice, she feels unseen and dismissed. She puts off coming back for years.

And she's not alone. What looks like "just one bad visit" adds up to a national crisis. A recent study found that avoidable deaths are rising in the United States, even as they fall across peer nations. Between 2009 and 2021, the United States saw an average increase of 32.5 avoidable deaths per 100,000 people, while European Union countries saw a decrease of 25.2.

In the following sections, I highlight ways in which the current system in the United States fails to take that "whole person" view, and how much patients lose when medicine refuses to connect the dots.

## *Holistic Health: Missing Connections*

Holistic health is an approach that considers the full person, not just isolated symptoms or diagnoses. It recognizes that physical, emotional, mental, and social factors are deeply interconnected, and that real healing requires addressing those layers together. But Western medicine in the United States isn't built this way. Instead, it tends to divide the body into specialties, reduce care to lab values and prescriptions, and overlook the broader context of a person's life.

This is where the system so often falls short: in seeing and helping the whole person. For example, a patient with PCOS likely needs much more than a medication recommendation. They may also need support with stress, movement, mental health, and sustainable lifestyle changes. But providers trained in silos often miss those needs entirely.

Western medicine focuses on what's "abnormal": irregular periods, elevated labs, an ultrasound result. Meanwhile other things go unnoticed, untreated, or referred out. When we fail to recognize how these parts connect, we don't just miss opportunities for better care, we leave patients carrying the burden of making sense of it all on their own. Patients are left trying to manage a complex condition while also piecing together care from different providers, none of whom are talking to each other.

Here's the key difference: holistic health is a *mindset*. It's about how we see the patient, as a whole person whose health is shaped by every layer of their life. It doesn't prescribe a specific therapy on its own; it's the lens through which care should be delivered.

## *Complementary, Integrative, and Functional Medicine: The Dismissed Toolbox*

When patients bring up acupuncture, herbal support, chiropractic care, or other complementary therapies, many clinicians are laced with doubt. Add functional medicine into the mix, a model that tries to trace symptoms back to root causes like hormone imbalance, inflammation, or nutritional gaps, and the skepticism only grows.

Instead of responding with curiosity and informed guidance, many providers are taught to dismiss what they don't recognize. That reflex doesn't just end a conversation; it tells the patient their experience isn't valid, especially if they've found it helpful. And that kind of dismissal quietly chips away at trust.

This disconnect is particularly problematic because so many patients already use complementary therapies, integrative approaches, or functional frameworks alongside conventional care, and often don't tell their providers. Without open, informed dialogue, patients are left navigating safety and efficacy alone.

And actually, medical students and faculty want this training. Surveys show strong interest in learning about complementary and integrative health, but the formal curricula just doesn't include it. For example, a survey at the Uniformed Services University of the Health Sciences found that 65% of students and 61% of faculty believed a complementary and integrative health curriculum should be instituted, yet it still hasn't been meaningfully integrated into medical education. Even with demand from both learners and educators, most medical schools still don't teach it in a comprehensive way. This leaves a glaring gap between what patients are doing, what providers want to know, and what the system delivers.

And that's not just an individual knowledge gap, it's a structural one. Successfully integrating complementary, integrative, and functional medicine into medical training requires more than a token elective or a guest lecture. It takes dedicated faculty, visible clinical practices, institutional investment, ongoing research, and a culture that treats these approaches as legitimate, not fringe. Without that foundation, these models of care stay optional, fragmented, and easy to dismiss, when they should be part of how we train providers to care for the whole person.

When providers can't engage with these approaches knowledgeably, they miss critical opportunities to prevent harmful interactions, validate helpful practices, and support patients' autonomy in choosing care that aligns with their values. The interesting thing? Some integrative therapies actually *do* have a strong evidence base: acupuncture for fertility, certain herbs for menstrual irregularities, and mindfulness for chronic pain. And functional medicine, for all its controversy, often overlaps with the very things patients are already asking about: nutrition, gut health, thyroid testing, environmental exposures.

In other words, these conversations are already happening. Patients are left piecing it together on their own instead of getting safe, informed guidance and unified care plans from the people they're supposed to be able to trust most.

### *Nutrition: A Missing Ingredient of Reproductive Care*

Despite nutrition directly affecting fertility, pregnancy outcomes, hormonal health, and chronic conditions like PCOS or insulin resistance, most OB-GYNs receive almost no training on how to counsel patients about food. In a 2023 survey of more than 1,000 US medical students, nearly 6 in 10 said they had received no formal nutrition education at all. Fewer than 8% had received 20 hours or more, still short of the recommended 25-hour minimum. And even within those limited hours, the focus was largely on biochemistry, not real-world, culturally relevant, or patient-centered nutrition counseling.

The consequences show up everywhere. Patients with PCOS are told to "just lose weight" without any concrete guidance on managing insulin resistance. People struggling with infertility rarely receive evidence-based nutrition support, despite growing research showing that certain dietary patterns may improve pregnancy rates. Prenatal nutrition advice is often limited to "take a prenatal vitamin," "don't drink," and "avoid sushi." It's hardly comprehensive, and barely useful for anyone, let alone patients navigating real-life challenges like food insecurity, nausea, or dietary restrictions.

Basic questions go unanswered. How much protein is actually needed during pregnancy? Which supplements are helpful versus harmful? What about food aversions, cultural dietary practices, or disordered eating? Most providers are flying blind—relying on outdated scripts or generic handouts that fail to address individual needs, preferences, or medical history.

And for patients in larger bodies, nutrition counseling is often laced with shame. Instead of receiving personalized care, they're told, explicitly or implicitly, that their body size is the problem. That their weight alone explains irregular periods, difficulty conceiving, or poor outcomes. That no matter the question, the answer is "lose weight." This isn't just ineffective, it's harmful.

When patients are shamed about their weight, they're less likely to seek care, more likely to withhold information, and at higher risk for both physical and mental health complications. And when care is delayed, dismissed, or filtered through bias, it doesn't just feel dehumanizing, it *is* dehumanizing.

But bias doesn't only harm people in bigger bodies. Underweight patients often slip under the radar because their size is seen as "healthy" or even ideal. That can mean missed conversations about nutrient deficiencies, eating disorders, or the impact of low body mass index on fertility, bone density, and pregnancy outcomes. Both ends of the spectrum are overlooked in different ways: one group shamed, the other neglected.

We need to stop treating weight as a moral failure, and start treating it like the complex, multifactorial, deeply personal topic it is. That means asking thoughtful questions instead of making assumptions. It means recognizing that not all weight gain is unhealthy, not all weight loss is helpful, and not all bodies need to be fixed.

If a provider hasn't been trained to understand how weight, nutrition, metabolism, hormones, and systemic bias intersect, they'll keep offering the same vague, judgmental advice. And patients will keep walking out of appointments feeling unseen.

### *Environmental Health: Hidden Hazards Around Us*

We don't talk nearly enough about how the world around us affects our reproductive health. Pesticides in our produce. Industrial air pollution in our neighborhoods. Endocrine-disrupting chemicals like bisphenol A (BPA), per- and polyfluoroalkyl substances (PFAS), and phthalates found in plastics, cosmetics, cookware, and packaging. Heavy metals in our drinking water. These aren't rare exposures, they're everyday ones.

Some of the most concerning are endocrine disruptors, which are chemicals that interfere with how our hormones function. They can overstimulate hormone receptors, block them, or change how hormones are produced and used in the body. BPA, for example, is still found in many food containers and water bottles, with studies showing traces in more than 90% of urine samples tested by the Centers for Disease Control.

PFAS, often called *forever chemicals*, are in food packaging, cookware, carpets, even some menstrual products, and have been linked to kidney, testicular, and breast cancers. Phthalates are used in personal care products like hair straighteners, dyes, shampoos, and perfumes. Some studies have tied frequent use of these products to higher risks of hormone-sensitive cancers, particularly among Black women, who are more likely to be exposed.

To be clear, the science isn't always definitive. As oncologist Mikkael Sekeres explained in a *Washington Post* op-ed, the evidence linking most of these chemicals to cancer is not nearly as strong as risks like smoking or alcohol. But the ubiquity of these exposures and the early signals linking them to fertility challenges, miscarriage, earlier menopause, and certain cancers make them impossible to ignore. Even if the absolute risks are small, they add up when nearly everyone is exposed, every day, for decades.

Here's the problem: when patients read about this research and bring it up in the exam room, they're often made to feel like they're overreacting or like they've fallen down some internet rabbit hole. And to be fair, many clinicians *do* get understandably frustrated when patients arrive with long lists of Google searches, worried about every chemical, food, or product they've ever touched. But that frustration exists partly because providers themselves haven't been trained in how to weigh these risks or communicate about them. It's not always that doctors don't care; it's that they're juggling so many urgent demands that environmental health falls to the bottom of the list. And when it's not part of standard training, it's easy for it to get pushed aside.

The result? The questions don't get asked. The advice isn't given. And the quiet, invisible, yet accumulating risks go unnoticed. Patients are left to wonder if something in their environment might be affecting their body. Providers are left unequipped to help.

## Forces Beyond the Clinic Walls

Reproductive healthcare isn't shaped only by what happens in the exam room. Economics, policy, and politics set the stage, determining who can access care, who can afford it, and even which providers are trained to deliver it.

### *Economic Realities: When Healthcare Is Out of Reach*

A patient needs a $300 medication but earns $12 an hour. Another skips follow-up appointments because missing work means missing rent. A third delays treatment for months, waiting for insurance approval that may never come. These aren't edge cases, they're the norm in American healthcare.

Dissecting the larger forces that make US healthcare so expensive is beyond the scope of this book. What I'm focusing on instead is the downstream reality: providers are tasked with caring for patients inside a system that routinely sets them up to fail. Most receive little to no training on how to recognize or respond to these economic barriers. Clinical recommendations are made in a vacuum, based on ideal scenarios that don't reflect the day-to-day constraints patients live with.

Reproductive healthcare doesn't begin and end in the clinic. It's shaped by a patient's ability to afford medication, take time off work, find transportation, secure childcare, and navigate an insurance system that often works against them. These barriers are not incidental. They are central to whether care is truly accessible. And when they're ignored, the results show up in real time: a prescription that costs hundreds out-of-pocket, an appointment scheduled without regard for a patient's work schedule, a critical service delayed because of prior authorization. On paper, the care plan may be sound. In practice, it can be completely out of reach.

The consequences are devastating. Nearly 4 in 10 women have skipped or postponed getting healthcare they needed because of the cost. Patients delay care, abandon treatment, or go without altogether. Not because they don't want care, but because the system wasn't built with them in mind. And the truth is, the system itself is unsustainable.

How can it possibly accommodate real people's lives when, for example, the only ultrasound appointment available in the next eight days is at 2 p.m. on a workday? The unspoken message is that you should be grateful you even got an appointment at all. Never mind the lost wages, the childcare scramble, or the employer you'll have to negotiate with to make it happen. Instead of feeling supported, patients are left with resentment and exhaustion, navigating a system that demands their flexibility but offers none in return.

If we aim to deliver equitable reproductive healthcare, we must treat access as a core part of the clinical equation, not a separate issue to be solved elsewhere. Economic barriers are clinical barriers. And addressing them requires providers to be not just skilled, but system-aware, resource-informed, and willing to ask: is this plan truly accessible to the person in front of me?

## How Policy and Politics Shape the Pipeline

Changes in federal policy don't only affect patients, they reshape the training of the providers you'll one day see. Most medical schools and residency programs are closely tied to federal funding streams like Medicare and Medicaid. When that funding shifts, so do the opportunities for training in certain specialties, procedures, or patient populations.

Even outside of clinical training, changes to student loan policy can determine who can realistically pursue a medical career at all. If access to graduate loans tightens, students from lower-income backgrounds may have to alter their career plans or choose shorter, less costly training paths. This is not because their passion changed, but because the math no longer works.

The result? Policy decisions made far from the exam room can directly influence what's taught, who gets to learn it, and which communities will have access to those providers years down the road. That's why keeping an eye on healthcare policy isn't just about protecting care today, it's about shaping the care that will exist tomorrow.

## Advocating for Yourself

Now you know why your provider might not ask about trauma, or screen for depression, or offer real options for pain relief. Why they might shut down when you bring up sexual problems, gloss over menopause, or fall silent in the face of your grief after a miscarriage. It's not because they don't care. It's because the system doesn't value or reinforce this type of care.

It trains providers to prioritize procedures and crises, not conversations and connection. And then it keeps them rushing, room to room, patient to patient, without the time or support to slow down. Some may not even realize the harm they cause. Others do, but feel powerless to change it within the constraints of a system built for volume, not humanity.

And this knowledge changes everything. Instead of walking into appointments wondering *What's wrong with me?* you can ask, "What's wrong with this system?" Instead of leaving visits with the sense that something was missing but not knowing what, you can name the gaps in real time.

The system has taught providers that certain topics don't matter enough to learn. But when you walk into that room knowing what you need and asking for it anyway—that's how we start teaching the system differently. Because now you know that it doesn't have to be this way.

# Chapter 4

# Care Wasn't Built for Everyone

*Some People Aren't Just Falling Through the Cracks, They've Been Failed from the Beginning*

The healthcare system doesn't just struggle to listen. It was never designed to serve everyone in the first place. And that failure doesn't fall evenly. It lands harder on certain communities: by race, gender identity, income, weight, age, sexuality, and disability status. For too many people, inadequate care isn't an outlier. It's the default.

Bias in medicine isn't just a matter of bad attitudes, it's about who the system was built to serve. For anybody whose body fits outside of the medical default of white, thin, cisgender, and straight, care is rarely straightforward. It is marked by more barriers, fewer accommodations, and worse outcomes. These gaps aren't hypothetical. They're real, they're measurable, and they cost lives.

In the pages ahead, I'll dig into how these failures actually show up, not in theory, but in real people's lives. Black women facing staggering maternal mortality rates. LGBTQ+ patients searching for providers who won't flinch at their pronouns. Patients in larger bodies dismissed before the exam even starts. Youth, elders, immigrants, disabled patients. All are navigating a system that treats them as an afterthought. The details differ, but the pattern is the same: healthcare wasn't built with them in mind.

## Black Women and the Burden of Bias

One statistic says it all. Black women in the United States are about three times more likely to die from pregnancy-related causes than white women. And no, this isn't just about poverty, education, or whether someone takes prenatal vitamins. Black maternal mortality, for example, is sometimes mischaracterized as the result of personal failings: poverty, education, or "lifestyle choices." But even when you control for those factors, the disparity remains. Centers for Disease Control data show that a Black woman with a college degree or higher is still more likely to die during pregnancy or childbirth than a white woman with less than a high school education.

It's not about lifestyle. It's not about self-advocacy. It's about systemic racism. Consider the story of Kaitlyn Joshua, a mother from Louisiana who miscarried at 11 weeks but was turned away from two emergency rooms because doctors feared prosecution under the state's abortion ban. She was left bleeding heavily, in pain, and terrified for her life. All because physicians worried that the standard treatment for miscarriage might be criminalized. It took her two full months to pass her miscarriage. As Joshua has since said, "What happened to me wasn't a fluke. It's what happens when abortion bans and racism collide in our hospitals. Black women are already dying at higher rates, and laws like these just stack the odds against us."

Patterns of structural exclusion and bias shape every level of care. For Black women, economic barriers and clinical gaps are often so tightly intertwined they can't be separated. In many regions, maternity providers are scarce, hospitals are closing, and obstetric services are stretched thin. Insurance coverage too often drops off during the critical postpartum period, just as support is most needed. Services like doulas, midwives, or lactation consultants remain harder to access, and the lack of racial diversity among clinicians further deepens the disconnect, despite evidence that representation improves outcomes. Layered together, these realities create dangerous conditions for pregnancy and postpartum care for Black women.

And some blind spots can be literally connected to skin color. A 2018 study of medical textbooks found that nearly 75% of images showed light skin, and fewer than 5% showed dark skin. That means many clinicians are never taught how common conditions look on Black patients. Rashes, infections, or inflammation can be missed or misdiagnosed. And when complications like blood clots or hemorrhage arise, delays aren't just about what can be seen on the surface. They're also about whether clinicians have been taught to trust Black patients' descriptions of pain, shortness of breath, or symptoms that can't be seen at all.

The same is true for pain management. Disparities in pain medication don't stop at gender; they deepen with race. Black women in labor are significantly less likely to receive adequate pain relief, even when they ask for it directly. Decades of research show that false beliefs about biological differences between Black and white patients persist in medicine. Ideas that Black people have thicker skin, less sensitive nerve endings, or higher pain tolerance still exist. These myths, rooted in slavery and scientific racism, still influence clinical judgment today. Combine that with implicit bias and the chronic underrepresentation of Black patients in medical research and training materials, and you have a system where Black pain is routinely underestimated, undertreated, and dismissed.

And this isn't just about comfort. When pain goes untreated, it can drive blood pressure dangerously high, increase the risk of serious complications, and derail the critical recovery period after birth.

Black women deserve better. And this system has no excuse left for not delivering it.

## Women of Color: A Broader Pattern

The crisis doesn't stop with Black women. The term *women of color*, first coined in 1977 by Black feminist leaders as a solidarity identity, not a biological one, reminds us that while the details differ across groups, the throughline is the same: reproductive healthcare wasn't built with women of color in mind.

Indigenous women face some of the highest maternal mortality rates in the nation, often in rural communities stripped of maternity care. Latina patients are more likely to encounter gaps in coverage, bias, or a lack of culturally responsive care that delays treatment. Asian American and Pacific Islander women are often collapsed into a single category in data reporting, but that masks critical differences, like the higher gestational diabetes rates observed in South Asian women, and the elevated preterm birth risk seen among Pacific Islander women. And across immigrant communities broadly, language access and fear of discrimination remain barriers that can keep people from care.

The specifics vary but the pattern doesn't. Women of color are statistically more likely to deliver in underfunded hospitals, have their pain dismissed, and see their needs ignored in medical research and education. These are not isolated oversights. They are predictable outcomes of a system designed around a narrow default. For too many women of color, inadequate care isn't an outlier. It's the baseline.

## Cultural Competency: Beyond Translation Services

These inequities don't just show up in outcomes. They show up in the exam room, in how cultural identity is, or more often isn't, understood.

Too often, "cultural competency" in reproductive healthcare gets reduced to surface-level fixes: provide a translator, avoid offensive language, memorize a few cultural "facts." But that's not real competency. True care means understanding how a patient's cultural background, religious beliefs, and community values shape their experiences with pregnancy, contraception, childbirth, and loss.

When providers rely on gestures instead of doing the deeper work of building trust, confronting bias, and honoring lived experience, patients feel the consequences. They feel it when their concerns are dismissed, when their values are misunderstood, when they're treated like a checklist instead of a whole person.

It shows up in small but critical moments. In some communities, modesty norms call for same-gender providers or limited physical contact. Contraceptive counseling may need to acknowledge religious guidance or communal decision-making. Even expressions of pain and discomfort vary across cultures, yet too few providers are trained to recognize those differences, let alone respond to them appropriately.

The consequences are real. When pain isn't expressed in a "textbook" way, it's often ignored. When cultural or religious values shape medical decisions, they're often misunderstood. When people feel unseen, they're less likely to come back. For refugee and immigrant communities in particular, mistrust and fear of judgment create additional barriers. These delays can worsen birth outcomes and deepen inequities.

And here's the hard truth: it's not enough to say "we value diversity" while avoiding the structures that keep inequities in place. Even in leading public health journals, researchers have found the term *institutional racism* is rarely named, despite being a fundamental driver of disparities. When we fail to confront racism and cultural competence in training, providers fail to confront it in practice. The result is care that never moves past politeness into equity.

Additionally, language access is a cornerstone of cultural competency. When Spanish-language resources are removed from government or healthcare websites, patients lose more than convenience. They lose timely access to appointments, vital guidance, and benefits. This policy-level decision interacts with clinical care: patients may miss screenings, delay care, or feel alienated in environments that already struggle with trust. Cultural competency therefore cannot be limited to translation; it must address the broader structures that enable, or block, access.

What's needed isn't a one-off workshop. It's a shift. Patients have always known what research is just beginning to say, which is that memorizing lists doesn't build trust. What makes the difference is cultural humility, an ongoing commitment to listen, learn, and show up differently. Cultural humility reframes the provider's role from expert to partner. It asks clinicians to recognize power imbalances, to name the assumptions baked into their training, and to engage patients as people who know their own bodies and needs.

Because racial bias and culturally aware care aren't side issues. They're central to whether healthcare feels safe, respectful, and effective.

## LGBTQ+ Health: Rising Numbers, Minimal Training

A healthcare system that fails to account for the full spectrum of human experience is failing by design. And nowhere is that more evident than in how we train clinicians to care for LGBTQ+ patients.

In 2020, Gallup estimated that 5.6% of US adults identified as LGBTQ+. Just four years later, that number had climbed to 9.3%. Nearly 1 in 10 Americans now openly identifies as lesbian, gay, bisexual, transgender, or another non-heterosexual identity, which is *twice* as many as just a decade ago.

The surge is being driven by younger generations. In 2020, about 16% of Gen Z adults identified as LGBTQ+. By 2024, that figure had climbed to nearly 23%. Millennials rose too, from 9% to 12% over the same period. By contrast, only 2–3% of baby boomers and fewer than 2% of the Silent Generation identify as LGBTQ+. The generational gap is undeniable. Each new wave of adults is entering the healthcare system with greater visibility and different needs, yet medical training has barely budged to meet them.

Despite the growing numbers of LGBTQ+ patients, medical students receive a median of just five hours of training on LGBTQ+ health across all four years of medical school. That's less time than is spent on rare tropical diseases most providers will never encounter. The result is predictable: care that is not just outdated, but often clinically wrong. And at times openly biased or offensive.

Nearly 4 in 10 LGBTQ+ patients report discrimination in healthcare, and almost one in four avoid preventive care altogether, fearing mistreatment. Missed cancer screenings, untreated sexually transmitted infections, and delayed reproductive care are predictable consequences. They're the structural outcomes of a curriculum that still treats queer health as an afterthought.

### *Queer Oversights*

One place this neglect shows up most clearly is in OB-GYN care for queer women. Sexual health is still framed through a narrow lens. One where straight, cisgender women are the default. That leaves queer patients misinformed, underserved, and rarely asked the right questions. If you're not in a relationship with a man, the system often assumes you're not sexually active, or not at risk. As a result, critical conversations about STI prevention, barrier methods, and safe sex practices between women are almost entirely absent from both sex education and medical visits.

Even the few available tools, like dental dams or gloves, are rarely discussed, much less offered. There's a gap between what's assumed to be "safe" and what actually protects queer patients in real life. And outdated provider training only makes it worse. Many gynecologists were never taught how to counsel queer patients on the risks of human papillomavirus (HPV) transmission, bacterial vaginosis (BV) recurrence, or herpes exposure through skin-to-skin contact. That knowledge gap gets passed on to patients who are told they're "low risk" when what they really are is overlooked.

And then there's contraception. Too often, OB-GYNs assume that if you're sexually active, it must be with a male partner, and if you're not on birth control, you must be "irresponsible." No one stops to ask a basic question: is pregnancy even physiologically possible in the context of your relationship? Instead, queer patients are told they "should be on something," even when there's zero risk of pregnancy. That assumption isn't just inaccurate, it's alienating.

Queer patients deserve care that doesn't default to straight. That asks real questions instead of relying on outdated scripts. That treats sexual health like a conversation, not a checklist.

The disparities are especially stark in maternal health. In a 2022 study from the Association of American Medical Colleges, 83% of queer women reported complications during pregnancy and birth, compared with 63% of heterosexual women. Neither figure is acceptable, but a 20-point gap is staggering. More than half of queer women in the study said bias or discrimination directly shaped their care experiences.

These aren't minor differences, they are the result of systemic neglect. And when LGBTQ+ family planning is still filed under the outdated category of "infertility," as if there is no other framework for two women building a family, it sends a message that couldn't be clearer: your needs are not considered standard medicine.

That neglect shows up everywhere, from the clinic walls to the birth certificate forms. Couples describe walking into delivery wards lined only with images of white, heterosexual families, their own existence erased before they even see a provider. Non-birthing lesbian partners have been stopped at the doors of the delivery room or forced to be listed as "father" on their child's paperwork. These details may look like bureaucratic oversights, but for families in the most vulnerable moments of their lives, they are sharp reminders of exclusion and stigma.

And the cost isn't just emotional, it's physical. Research shows that queer women living in states with stronger legal protections for sexual minorities have measurably better birth outcomes: lower rates of preterm birth and higher birth weights, compared to those in states with fewer protections. Discrimination isn't just an unpleasant backdrop, it directly alters medical outcomes. Chronic stress, fear of mistreatment, and the constant burden of hiding or defending your identity manifest biologically as inflammation, immune dysfunction, and higher risks of complications.

This is something I carry with me every single day as a provider. In physician associate school, before my very first rotation, I pinned a small rainbow pride button onto my short student white coat. I've worn one every day I've practiced medicine since. Over the years, patients, queer and straight alike, have told me what that pin meant to them: safety, recognition, relief. A signal that they weren't invisible in the exam room.

When I pushed for basic changes like gender-inclusive intake forms, I was told it might "offend" other patients, that it wasn't worth the trouble. And then in 2021, I fought to add pronouns to our clinician bios online. A small step, maybe, but for patients who rarely see themselves reflected in clinical spaces, it mattered. And it mattered to me, too. That was the kind of clinician I wanted to be. Seeing and affirming people wasn't an add-on; it was core to my identity as a provider. Then, in fall 2024, on the day I was fired, my name and photo disappeared from the company website. And so did the pronouns.

This is why we have to stand up even louder. Because it's not only that progress isn't happening fast enough, it's that in some cases, we're watching hard-won changes disappear. For queer patients across the United States, it's not simply a matter of waiting for better care; it's seeing inclusion rolled back in ways that make healthcare feel less safe, less welcoming, and less trustworthy.

None of this should be controversial. Recognizing diverse families and identities isn't about politics. It's about accuracy, safety, and dignity. When patients see themselves reflected and respected, they are more likely to seek care, share critical details, and trust the medical system. That isn't ideology, it's just good medicine. The sooner we stop treating inclusion as optional, the sooner we begin closing the disparities that harm millions of people who simply want what every patient deserves: to be seen, heard, and cared for as they are.

### *The Transgender Healthcare Gap*

For transgender and gender nonconforming (TGNC) patients, even showing up for care can feel like a risk. A risk of being misgendered. A risk of being stared at. A risk of being denied care altogether. Nearly one in four transgender adults have avoided seeking care due to anticipated discrimination, and trans men face even higher rates of avoidance.

That avoidance doesn't come from not valuing their health. It comes from experience. Experience that tells them: this system wasn't built with you in mind.

Across the board, TGNC patients report high rates of misgendering, harassment, erasure, and outright denial of services. And new research confirms what trans patients have been saying for years: barriers to affirming, competent care remain the norm, from providers refusing gender-affirming care to gaps in insurance coverage and training.

So what's behind all this harm? Often, it's not overt cruelty, it's clinical ignorance. The most commonly cited barrier? A basic lack of knowledgeable providers. Most clinicians have never been trained in gender-affirming gynecological care. They don't know what questions to ask, or how to ask them without causing harm. They don't understand how hormone therapy intersects with cancer screening. They don't know how to offer trauma-informed pelvic exams for someone navigating gender dysphoria.

This isn't about feelings. It's about lifesaving access, because when you expect to be disrespected, you delay care. And when care is delayed, complications multiply. People miss cancer screenings. Infections go untreated. Reproductive decisions become limited, not by anatomy, but by the fear of being mistreated in the exam room.

Trans and nonbinary people deserve providers who know how to care for their bodies and affirm their identities. Not as an afterthought. Not as a one-off checkbox. As a standard.

Affirming care is not a niche specialty. It's basic human dignity. And it's long overdue.

## Weight as a Barrier to Care Access

> *Note: In this section, we use the word fat intentionally—not as an insult, but as a neutral, descriptive term, the way many fat activists and scholars use it. Terms like obese and overweight come from medical models that pathologize body size and frame fatness as a disease. That framing often contributes to the very stigma we're trying to unpack here.*

If you live in a larger body, you don't need research to know the system wasn't built with you in mind. But the numbers confirm it. In a national survey of healthcare facilities, 91% couldn't weigh patients over 350 pounds, 87% didn't stock gowns that fit, and nearly one in four lacked armless chairs, basic equipment that would signal patients belong in the room.

These aren't small oversights. They're architectural exclusions. And they send a message loud and clear: "We didn't plan for you to be here. We didn't prioritize your comfort."

I saw this firsthand in the clinic where I worked. It had been open for over 40 years, and in all that time, I was the only provider who had ever requested that we stock larger gowns. The only clinician who consistently used them. My medical assistants would often reach for the standard size, even when it was visibly too small for the patient in front of them. And I'd step in. Because it's a simple thing, really, offering a gown that actually fits.

But it matters. It tells the patient, "You belong here. I see you." Without it, that gown might as well be a napkin folded across your lap. I never wanted my patients to feel degraded or self-conscious like that. I wanted them to feel cared for. Respected. And that starts before a single word is spoken.

But in my workplace, speaking up about it made me the problem. Correcting a medical assistant for handing over a gown that wouldn't fit wasn't seen as advocating for patients, it was seen as me being difficult. Demanding. *Too much.* In a system that normalizes discomfort for fat patients, insisting on dignity was treated as disruption.

And the truth is, it's not just about gowns or equipment. Weight stigma among health professionals shows up in both explicit and implicit ways. Studies show that physicians spend less time with higher-weight patients, provide fewer preventive services, and offer less health education compared to thinner patients. Clinicians often assume fat patients are lazy, noncompliant, or uninterested in their health. Those assumptions derail everything, from the seriousness with which a concern is taken to whether a condition is even diagnosed.

The impact is devastating. Research shows that weight stigma leads to fewer cancer screenings, skipped prenatal visits, and delayed general care. In one study, 21% of patients said they would change doctors entirely if they felt judged for their weight. Others avoid care altogether, not because they don't value their health, but because they've learned the exam room often means walking into judgment.

And stigma doesn't just hurt emotionally, it harms biologically. Independent of body size, experiencing weight discrimination is linked to higher cortisol levels, systemic inflammation, and increased cardiometabolic risk. In other words, stigma itself makes people sicker. The cruel irony is that shame doesn't reduce weight; in fact, longitudinal studies show that people who experience weight discrimination are more likely to gain weight over time.

This is why leading researchers now argue that freedom from weight discrimination should be recognized as a fundamental human right. Until medicine stops treating fat bodies as problems to be solved and starts treating them as people to be cared for, weight will remain a barrier not only to dignity but to health itself.

## Youth and Adolescents: Treated Like They Don't Belong Yet

Young people, especially teens ages 13 to 19, are often treated as though they don't belong in the exam room at all. Adolescents too often enter spaces designed to monitor their behavior, not meet their needs. They're met with judgment, discomfort, or silence. Their questions are brushed off, their needs delayed, and their rights, when they have them, are rarely explained.

Depending on the state, teens may or may not be able to consent to their own reproductive healthcare. They may be required to notify or get permission from a parent before accessing birth control, emergency contraception, STI testing, or abortion care. Even in places where youth have legal rights to confidential services, providers don't always explain those rights, nor offer an environment where young people feel safe using them.

And while schools may claim to provide health education, most students graduate without ever learning how to recognize normal versus abnormal symptoms, how to navigate a pelvic exam, or how to advocate for themselves in a medical setting. In fact, many teens still believe that a Pap smear is required to get birth control, or that a pelvic exam is standard at every visit. They learn that from outdated curricula, and sometimes from the clinics themselves.

Then there's the provider side. Far too many OB-GYNs were never properly trained to care for adolescents. They may speak down to them. They may assume heterosexual activity. They may shame a teen for seeking contraception or STI testing. Or they may avoid asking about sex or relationships altogether out of discomfort, leaving young people to figure it out on their own.

And when a young person walks in with a parent or guardian, it gets even trickier. The default is often to direct all questions to the adult, leaving the actual patient silent in the corner. But care that isn't youth-centered fails to serve the person most at risk of being left out.

It's also worth saying: not every teen has affirming or safe adults in their life. For LGBTQ+ youth, immigrant teens, young people in foster care, or those experiencing abuse or neglect, that adult in the room might not be a source of support. It might be the barrier. Which means it's up to the provider to create a safe, confidential space where real care can happen.

When we delay or deny gynecologic care for young people, we don't just increase their medical risk we also reinforce the idea that their questions, their bodies, and their needs don't matter yet. That's not just bad practice. It's dangerous.

Young people don't need to wait until they're older to be taken seriously. They need, and deserve, care that's trauma-informed, shame-free, and built on their right to know, ask, and advocate. Because the sooner someone learns to trust their body and their voice, the more likely they are to carry that trust with them—for a lifetime.

## Midlife and Beyond: Treated Like You've Aged Out

Imagine walking into the doctor's office with new pain, brain fog, or sleepless nights, only to be told, "That's just menopause. That's just aging." For women in midlife and beyond, this isn't imagination. It's the reality of care that too often shrugs off real symptoms and writes off real experiences.

Ageism in healthcare is everywhere, and it takes a real toll. One national study found that more than 9 out of 10 adults between 50 and 80 had experienced everyday ageism, and those experiences were directly tied to worse physical and mental health. And it's not just in the United States, a global review of hundreds of studies across 45 countries found the same pattern: in the vast majority, ageism was linked to worse health outcomes. People received fewer tests, fewer referrals, or were even denied treatments, not because they didn't need them, but because the system had quietly decided they'd "aged out" of care.

Even communication changes. Reviews of research show that clinicians often interact differently with patients in later life: physicians may be less patient, less respectful, and less engaged in care conversations, while nurses spend less time, offer more superficial explanations, and lean on ageist stereotypes during appointments.

By the time women reach the postmenopause years, the pattern is familiar: their symptoms are minimized, their needs overlooked. Between 50 and 65, this neglect can be especially dangerous—when hot flashes, brain fog, and sexual changes persist, bone loss accelerates, and cardiovascular risks begin to climb. Yet many stop seeing their OB-GYN once periods and pregnancies are behind them, and primary care providers too often fail to step in. That gap leaves countless women in the postmenopause years without support during the very stage when treatment could make the most difference.

And it doesn't stop at the clinic door. The same ageism that dismisses women's health in midlife and postmenopause shows up everywhere: in advertising, in workplaces, and even in relationships. The culture reflects back the same message as the clinic: that once fertility ends, women's bodies, and their experiences, are somehow less important. Beauty and wellness industries center on youth, while real conversations about what it feels like to live in a changing body are sidelined. The result is that women carry double the weight: symptoms that go untreated and a culture that tells them those symptoms make them irrelevant.

But the truth is, women in their 50s, 60s, and beyond are at the height of their leadership, influence, and wisdom. They are raising teenagers, young adults, and sometimes grandchildren, running companies, shaping communities, falling in love again, reimagining themselves. The disconnect between that reality and the silence they encounter in healthcare isn't just frustrating, it's damaging. It reinforces the idea that midlife is an ending, when in fact it's often the most powerful chapter yet.

And in gynecology, the message is especially clear: once you turn 65, you've aged out of relevance. Many OB-GYN offices don't even accept Medicare, the primary insurance for people in their postmenopause years. Not because those patients don't need care, but because the system has quietly decided they're no longer worth accommodating. Even the guidelines reinforce the idea that aging means irrelevance: if your Pap smears have been normal, cervical cancer screening is officially recommended to stop at 65.

From a cancer-prevention standpoint, that can be reasonable, especially if you remain low-risk without new exposures. But the unspoken message is damaging. It suggests patients are "done" being seen, when in reality they may still need pelvic exams, urinary tract infection treatment, prolapse care, hormone support, or space to talk openly about sex, pain, or urinary changes.

This silence is especially glaring when it comes to menopause care. For decades, women have been told that hormone therapy must be stopped at 65, that their window has closed, that symptoms are simply their new normal. But the evidence doesn't support a blanket cutoff. Guidelines now emphasize that if someone began hormone therapy earlier and is still benefiting, there is no rule that it must be discontinued just because they've hit a birthday. For some, the risks do increase with age. But for many, individualized decisions—balancing bone health, sexual comfort, sleep, and quality of life—are far safer than the blanket dismissal that has become the norm.

People don't stop having bodies at 65, and they certainly don't stop having sex. In fact, many reenter their sexual lives in new ways after divorce, widowhood, or decades in one relationship. Some are exploring intimacy with new partners for the first time in years. Some are coming out later in life. But almost none are being asked about it in the exam room.

Sexual health for those in midlife and beyond isn't just under-discussed, it's almost entirely ignored. That silence carries risk. STIs are surprisingly prevalent in senior communities and nursing homes, precisely because no one's talking about prevention. No one's offering condoms, discussing barrier options, or screening routinely. In fact, older adults are now the second-highest group for new HIV and syphilis diagnoses after college-age youth.

This stage of life isn't a curtain call. It's decades of living, working, loving, leading, reinventing. Healthcare should rise to meet that, not disappear when the hot flashes fade. Being postmenopausal should never mean being dismissed.

## Disability as Deficiency

People with disabilities make up nearly one in six people globally. In the United States, they represent about 27% of adults but account for roughly 36% of all healthcare spending. Yet disabled people often encounter inaccessible spaces, ill-informed providers, and a medical system that views their existence as something to be "fixed."

This isn't just about physical access, though that matters deeply. Studies show that the majority of healthcare settings lack basic accessible equipment such as height-adjustable exam tables, wheelchair-accessible scales, or transfer devices. Imagine needing a Pap smear or an annual exam and realizing the table can't even lower to accommodate your wheelchair. That's not just uncomfortable, it's exclusion in action.

But barriers aren't only physical. Many disabilities are invisible—chronic pain, autoimmune disorders, neurological conditions, mental health diagnoses—and these patients often face disbelief, minimization, or outright dismissal. If a provider can't "see" the disability, they may assume it isn't real, or they may treat the patient as exaggerating. That invisibility compounds stigma and delays care just as much as inaccessible exam tables.

And bias runs deep. In one study of US healthcare providers, 76% reported positive attitudes toward patients with disabilities, yet 84% simultaneously showed strong implicit bias against them. The authors categorized most participants as "aversive ableists," people who say the right things out loud but still hold hidden prejudice. That kind of bias is especially dangerous because it hides behind good intentions.

It results in assumptions that disabled people don't need gynecological care. That they don't need contraception. That they aren't sexually active. That they can't parent. That their concerns are just "part of their condition." And that they won't understand what's being said, so there's no point explaining in full.

When disability, visible or invisible, is seen as deficiency, patients are treated like a problem to manage, not a person to care for. And that's the real failure: not disability itself, but a system that refuses to accommodate, affirm, and honor disabled lives.

## Rural and Low-Income Communities

In rural areas, OB-GYN care can be hours away, if it exists at all. Entire counties have no practicing obstetric providers, and in more than half of US rural counties, there's no hospital offering labor and delivery services. These maternity care deserts have only expanded over the last decade, driven by hospital closures, financial strain, and persistent provider shortages.

Even when a clinic is nearby, cost and coverage can still shut the door. Nationally, nearly 8 in 10 OB-GYN practices accept Medicaid. But access isn't equal everywhere. OB-GYNs are heavily concentrated in metropolitan and higher-income areas, leaving many rural counties without a single provider. Rural OB-GYNs are actually more likely to accept Medicaid, but the scarcity of providers means patients still face a double barrier: too few clinics within reach and too many stretched thin or not accepting new patients.

For low-income patients, delays don't just mean waiting, they mean going without. Clinic closures and abortion restrictions disproportionately affect rural communities, where transportation is limited, child care is expensive, and time off work isn't guaranteed. When care is too far, too costly, or too complicated to reach, people delay, or don't go at all.

And the consequences are stark. People in rural and low-income areas experience higher rates of preventable pregnancy complications, delayed prenatal care, and higher maternal mortality, not because of personal choices, but because of policy-driven access gaps. The safety net that rural hospitals and patients rely on, Medicaid, is perpetually vulnerable to political cuts and restrictions. Each new proposal to scale it back threatens to deepen the strain on communities already struggling to access care.

Healthcare deserts don't just appear on their own, they're the result of political choices and systemic neglect. Unless those choices change, the very structures meant to provide care will continue to erode, leaving communities even more deserted than they are today.

## Immigrant and Non-English-Dominant Patients

For immigrant and undocumented patients, showing up to a clinic can feel risky. Not because they don't value their health but because they've learned the system doesn't always protect it. Fear of being reported, dismissed, or mistreated keeps many from accessing OB-GYN care until it's urgent. Add in limited or no insurance coverage, and the barriers only grow.

Language can make or break the experience. Patients who don't primarily speak English, or who feel more comfortable in another language, face serious risks in medical settings. Without trained interpreters, patients are left to guess what's happening. Consent forms go untranslated. Diagnoses are misunderstood.

Patients nod along not because they agree, but because they're scared or unsure how to ask questions.

And this isn't rare: nearly 25 million people in the United States speak a language other than English at home and report difficulty communicating in healthcare settings. Yet one study found that only 13% of hospitals met all four standards for linguistically appropriate care, and 19% met none at all.

Even patients who can navigate English in everyday conversation often struggle with the jargon-heavy, high-stakes language of medicine. Assumptions like "they seem fine" or "they understand enough" can lead to real harm. This isn't about fluency, it's about safety. Language access isn't a bonus feature. It's foundational to ethical, informed, patient-centered care.

## A Dangerous Overlap: When Identities Intersect

Any of these factors—race, disability, gender identity, weight, age, income—can shape how you're treated in a medical setting. But when they intersect? The harm doesn't just add up. It multiplies. Black and fat. Trans and disabled. Old and low-income. The more your identity diverges from the medical "default," the more likely you are to be overlooked, mistreated, or written off entirely.

And for those at the intersection of multiple marginalized identities, the system's failures aren't just more frequent, they're more dangerous. Not because of who they are, but because of how little the system was ever built to see them.

# Chapter 5

# The Illusion of Coverage

*How Insurance Turns Access into an Obstacle Course*

In reproductive healthcare, it's not just what your provider knows, it's what they're allowed to do. And in America, what they're allowed to do is dictated, more than anything, by insurance.

Here's what that actually means in practice: your provider only gets paid for services they can bill to your insurance company. And they can only bill for services that have an approved billing code. If there's no code for something, it's like it doesn't exist in the system, no matter how important it is to your care.

Those billing codes don't just describe what gets done, they decide how much it's worth. And the system values some things far more than others. Procedures, surgeries, and diagnostic tests get higher reimbursement rates. Counseling, mental health screening, or just taking time to explain your options? Those are undervalued, or not reimbursed at all.

Why not just do those things anyway? Some providers try. But the reality is, they still have to see a certain number of patients a day to keep the clinic running. If they spend extra time on an unpaid service, it means running behind, cutting into someone else's visit, or losing the income that keeps the doors open. If they do it too often, they risk being labeled "inefficient" by administrators, which can affect their pay, or their job.

Insurance shapes every corner of care. It determines who gets in the door, how long visits last, what gets discussed, what gets reimbursed, and what's deemed "medically necessary." It doesn't follow clinical best practices, it follows billing codes and reimbursement rules. If something can't be coded, it often doesn't happen.

What results is a version of care that prioritizes what insurance will pay for—not what you actually need.

## Undervalued at Every Level

Until recently, billing was mostly tied to procedures and diagnoses in healthcare. "Billing by time" exists now, but it's rarely practical. The documentation burden is high, reimbursement is inconsistent, and it still doesn't account for emotional labor or education. Productivity is tracked using relative value units—the medical system's price tags. They put a number on every task your provider does. The more complex or invasive the procedure, the higher the number, and the more it's worth. Surgeries and high-tech imaging rack up points quickly. But conversations? Counseling? Mental health screening? They barely register.

This is especially true in OB-GYN care, where time-intensive services like counseling, miscarriage support, or mental health screening don't carry the same financial "value" as a procedure. The system rewards procedures, not presence. Conversations don't generate revenue. Holding space for grief or explaining options thoroughly? There's no line item for that. Emotional labor doesn't get documented.

The payment system systematically undervalues cognitive services—counseling, education, and shared decision-making—while rewarding procedures, even though these conversations are the backbone of quality reproductive care. A provider can spend 20 minutes walking a patient through birth control options, clarifying side effects, and making sure the final choice feels right, and still be reimbursed far less than they would for inserting an intrauterine device (IUD) in a quarter of the time. The result is a distorted incentive structure: listening, teaching, and partnering with patients—the very elements that build trust and ensure safe, effective care—are treated as less valuable than quick interventions.

And if there isn't a current procedural terminology (CPT) code for what you're talking about, a five-digit number used for reimbursement, it's as if that interaction never happened, leaving the education and emotional labor that shape outcomes invisible and uncompensated. Some providers still try to sneak those moments in because they know it matters. But the system punishes them for it. Run too long and you get dinged, do it too often and you're labeled inefficient.

Even within procedures and surgeries themselves, gynecology loses out. Because who decides what those codes are worth? Not always the people doing the work. In fact, the national committees that assign value to procedures often don't include gynecologic surgeons. That means office-based OB-GYNs who may never perform advanced surgery are still voting on how much those surgeries should pay. Unsurprisingly, the result is that gynecologic procedures are undervalued, access shrinks, and patients are told their options are limited. One *JAMA Surgery* commentary described this dynamic as a structural barrier that keeps women's health perpetually underfunded.

## Bundled Payments and Value-Based Care

Another insurance "innovation," ostensibly meant to control costs, has made things even harder: bundled payments and value-based care.

In a bundled payment system, the provider (or the healthcare organization they work for) gets a single lump sum from the insurance company to cover all the care for a certain condition or time period, like an entire pregnancy, birth, and postpartum period. That lump sum is meant to pay for *everything* in that package, from routine prenatal visits to the delivery itself to any standard postpartum visits in the first six weeks.

On paper, these models are supposed to reward good outcomes rather than sheer volume of services. But in OB-GYN, they're often detrimental. A "bundled" maternity payment, for example, might include all prenatal care, labor, delivery, and the standard six-week postpartum visit in one flat fee. That sounds efficient. That is until a patient needs extra monitoring for high blood pressure, extra appointments for pregnancy after loss, or more than one postpartum check-in.

Bundled payment models create a troubling math problem: when pregnancies need care beyond the standard package, providers often absorb the cost without additional compensation. The system assumes pregnancies fit neatly into predictable boxes. When someone needs extra monitoring, more frequent visits, or intensive support for complications, the economics quietly infiltrate every clinical decision.

This isn't always a conscious calculation. Even well-meaning providers operate within financial constraints that become embedded in their clinical reasoning. The payment can stay the same whether a pregnancy is straightforward or requires weeks of additional management, and that reality doesn't just influence explicit resource allocation. It subtly steers clinical judgment toward interventions that fit within the reimbursed framework. In practice, providers are effectively paid less per hour for the very patients who need the most, creating an economic undertow that pulls against intensive, individualized care.

It's why your prenatal care is often scheduled in those rigid every four weeks, then every two weeks, then weekly intervals, whether or not you'd benefit from being seen more often. It's why if you have anxiety in pregnancy and ask to come in just to hear the fetal heart tones, you might be met with resistance, told "that's not necessary," or asked to wait until your next scheduled appointment. The system isn't built for what reassures you, it's built for what fits the payment model. Providers are reimbursed for a set amount of care, and that framework dictates the schedule more than your individual needs.

This is also why postpartum care in the United States is so bare bones. Since the early postpartum period is included in that single global payment, there's no additional reimbursement for seeing a new parent more than once in those first six weeks. That's why so many people get only one postpartum check, and why serious issues—like high blood pressure, wound complications, breastfeeding struggles, or mental health concerns—can go undetected until they become emergencies.

Mental health screening is a perfect example. Simple questionnaires like the PHQ-9, a two-minute depression screening tool, are widely recommended during postpartum and routine visits. Yet they're often excluded from reimbursement. Research consistently shows that systematic postpartum depression screening could not only improve quality of life but also prevent significant numbers of maternal deaths by suicide. Despite this evidence, most OB-GYN practices don't consistently use standardized screening tools, not because they don't work or because providers don't believe in them, but because the time spent administering and interpreting them isn't billable. Two minutes that could save a life becomes two minutes that costs the practice money, and the math speaks for itself.

At my last practice, I pleaded for our team to add the PHQ-9 to our six-week postpartum visits. In my mind it wasn't a radical ask, it was the bare minimum. A two-minute depression screening tool. Even my own child's pediatrician handed me one when I brought my baby in for their one-month checkup, because they understood that a parent's mental health is essential to a child's well-being.

And here's what makes that so striking: pediatricians aren't there for the moms. They don't manage postpartum recovery. They're not reimbursed for maternal health. Their entire job is to make sure the baby is growing, feeding, thriving. But still, they paused long enough to see me, too. To acknowledge that my well-being mattered because my child's depended on it.

Meanwhile, when I asked my own OB-GYN team to do the same for our patients, the pushback was immediate. The answer wasn't about clinical need or best practice. It was, "We don't get paid for it." And worse, "You could open up a can of worms that you don't have time to manage."

That told me everything. Not that the screening lacked value, but that a mother's suffering was treated as expendable the moment it didn't come with a billing code.

### The Access Lottery

Who you are, and what kind of insurance you carry, shapes your access to care. About one in four doctors won't take new Medicaid patients, even though Medicaid covers more than 40% of births in the United States. And that lack of access doesn't fall evenly. Only about a quarter of white mothers give birth on Medicaid, but for Hispanic mothers it's more than half, and for Black mothers it's nearly two-thirds. The result is a system where access isn't evenly distributed. When providers step away from Medicaid, it's women of color, and their babies, who lose access.

Medicaid pays providers far less than private insurance, which makes it harder for many clinics to keep their doors open to those patients. And when fewer doctors accept Medicaid, the problem compounds in rural communities where providers are scarce to begin with. In those areas, the access gap is even sharper: only about 7% of OB providers practice in rural communities, even though more than half a million babies are born there each year. That leaves families driving hours for basic prenatal visits, with fewer choices once they arrive. Layer racial disparities on top of that geography gap, and the picture gets even starker. Women of color are more likely to live in maternity care deserts, places with no hospital offering obstetric care and no OB-GYN or midwife within reach.

For families living in these deserts, the promise of telemedicine feels obvious. Telemedicine could help bridge some of these gaps: shortening wait times, reducing travel, and expanding access in communities where there are no nearby providers. A virtual visit can't replace every aspect of prenatal or gynecologic care, but it can cover a lot: counseling, prescription management, postpartum check-ins, mental health screenings, contraceptive care, even some early pregnancy visits. For people who live hours from the nearest OB-GYN, or who can't easily arrange childcare or time off work, telehealth can mean the difference between getting care and going without.

But even where virtual care could make a difference, the policies governing it fall short. Reimbursement rules vary wildly and rarely cover what's needed. Some insurers still don't reimburse for remote visits at all, despite expanded use during the pandemic. Many state policies require in-person visits for things that could be done virtually, and only a minority of state Medicaid programs allow patients to receive covered telehealth services from home, creating more barriers for those with limited transportation or childcare.

And behind it all is a bigger problem: getting an appointment in the first place. Insurance doesn't just decide what gets paid for, it decides who gets seen, and how soon. The average wait time to see an OB-GYN is now more than 31 days. That's a full week longer than it was just a few years ago, a 19% jump since 2017. And that's only the average. In some places, especially rural and underserved areas, the wait stretches to four months or more. For women of color on Medicaid, in counties where the fewest providers participate, "wait time" often isn't measured in weeks at all. It looks like no appointment available, period.

In a country where nearly half of all births are paid for by Medicaid, access to care shouldn't come down to luck of geography, race, or insurance card. But right now, it does.

## The Cost of Care

Patients are often told their care is "covered." But that doesn't mean it's affordable. Copays, deductibles, out-of-pocket costs, and denied claims pile up fast. A prescription might technically be on your insurance company's "formulary," their official list of approved drugs, but still cost $100 at the pharmacy. An ultrasound might be approved, but only if it's billed under the right diagnosis code. A visit might be allowed, but not the actual conversation that happens during it.

And the burden doesn't stop at a few surprise fees. It piles up until it breaks people. Forty-one percent of US adults are carrying medical or dental debt. Nearly two-thirds of them *had insurance* when those bills came due. And of those insured patients, three-quarters said their copays, deductibles, or coinsurance were more than they could afford.

For women of reproductive age, the numbers cut even deeper: half report putting off or skipping needed care in the past year because of cost. That means skipped appointments, delayed tests, and prescriptions left unfilled, not because people didn't want the care, but because they couldn't afford it.

This is the impossible math of American healthcare. Do I refill my prescription or pay for gas? Do I make that doctor's appointment or make rent? For too many families, it isn't a question of convenience, it's a question of survival.

And then there are the costs that aren't covered at all.

Fertility treatments, even for patients with medical diagnoses like polycystic ovary syndrome (PCOS) or endometriosis, are often dismissed as "elective" and excluded from insurance coverage. Many plans will pay for testing to confirm infertility, but stop short of covering the treatments that follow. That leaves patients paying out of pocket for essential medical care. A single in vitro fertilization (IVF) cycle runs $12,000 to $20,000, and once you add medications, embryo storage, or genetic testing, the price can soar past $30,000. The average cycle costs $12,400, before any of those add-ons, and most women require multiple IVF cycles to achieve a live birth.

The financial toll is staggering. Seventy percent of women who undergo fertility treatment end up in debt, and nearly half borrow more than $10,000 to cover it. Four out of five couples report their finances were significantly strained, often draining savings or relying on credit to pay for care. And all of this for healthcare that's routinely labeled "optional," when for many, it's anything but.

Miscarriage care can carry similar financial trauma. A patient who needs an emergency dilation and curettage might receive a $5,000 bill, despite being told their care was "covered." Charges for the emergency room, anesthesia, pathology, or hospital facility fees often come separately and unexpectedly. Grief is already heavy. The financial aftermath only compounds it.

Coverage doesn't always mean protection. Too often, it means confusion. Loopholes you didn't know existed, denials that come out of nowhere, and bills that land weeks later with no explanation. And the fallout isn't just on patients. For providers, every billing battle is time stolen from actual care.

The administrative load is staggering. An American Medical Association survey found that physicians and their staff spend an average of 13 hours each week completing prior authorization requests, about 39 requests per physician, per week. Forty percent of doctors say they even have staff whose sole job is wrangling prior authorizations. Nearly 9 in 10 physicians report that the process fuels burnout, and more than a quarter say it has directly harmed patients: causing hospitalizations, life-threatening events, or even disability and death.

## When Problems Aren't Convenient

Take the annual exam. On paper, it's a "well-woman visit." That means it's preventative and covered. But only if nothing's wrong. If a patient brings up pain with sex, irregular bleeding, or postpartum depression? It becomes a problem visit. That changes the billing code, which often triggers partial reimbursement at best, and outright denials or audits at worst. So providers are discouraged, explicitly or implicitly, from addressing both prevention and problems in the same visit.

But research shows that patients typically present multiple complaints during office visits because it's often their only visit all year. And they have no idea how it all works. And if that visit runs long because of what comes up? That extra time is often unreimbursed. Research shows that physicians spend substantial time on work that is not explicitly reimbursed, including medical record review, documentation, and coordination of care, with many physicians reporting averaging one to two hours of unreimbursed, after-hours work daily. So patients either leave with unanswered questions or providers absorb the uncompensated time.

Some practices even train their front desk staff to give you the warning when you schedule your annual: "If you bring up any medical concerns, it might not be covered." It doesn't mean you can't ask questions. It just means you have to be strategic about *when* you ask them if you want the time, attention, and answers you deserve.

## The Cost of Medication

For too many patients, the real barrier isn't whether a treatment exists, it's whether the system will recognize it. In our insurance-based model, care only "counts" if it fits the right billing code, shows up on a formulary, or meets an insurer's definition of "medically necessary." If it doesn't, it might as well not exist.

That's why cost sharing and coverage rules so often block people from the medications they need. Even with Medicaid, 1 in 10 low-income women report leaving a prescription unfilled in the past year because of cost. In many states, that's because coverage comes with strings attached: caps on the number of prescriptions, limits on visits, or copayments for medications if you're a nonpregnant adult. Affordability barriers don't vanish under Medicaid—they just show up in new forms, even inside a program meant to remove them.

And for patients, these barriers aren't abstract, they're lived. Someone might be told their medication is covered, only to arrive at the pharmacy and be blindsided by a copay. Others are forced to "fail" on cheaper drugs first, even when those options have already caused side effects or simply don't work. In those moments, access isn't about what's medically best, it's about persistence, paperwork, or price.

## The Contraceptive Coverage Maze

Last year I had a patient who was thrilled to try a new kind of birth control. It used a different kind of estrogen, had a lower side-effect profile, and early studies showed people tolerated it better than traditional options. For her, it felt like hope after years of side effects from other methods. But the system shut her down. Her insurance wouldn't cover it. Local pharmacies didn't stock it. The prior authorization was denied without explanation. A method that could have improved her quality of life was suddenly out of reach. Not because it wasn't safe or effective, but because the system had already decided it wasn't worth it.

That's the reality with contraception in America. The Affordable Care Act requires most health insurance plans to cover contraception without cost sharing. On paper, that sounds simple. In practice, accessing the method you actually need is anything but. Insurers are only required to cover one option in each Food and Drug Administration (FDA)-defined contraceptive category. That means your plan might pay for a pill, but not the one that doesn't make you sick. It might cover a hormonal IUD, but not the copper one—or vice versa. Technically, you're "covered." In reality, you're not.

And even when the method you want is technically covered, insurers pile on the red tape: "fail first" rules that force patients to try cheaper methods first, prior authorizations for FDA-approved options, strict refill limits that send people back to the pharmacy again and again, and rigid formularies that ignore medical necessity. A 2023 analysis found that insurers denied about 40% of contraceptive coverage exception requests, blocking patients from accessing their preferred method of birth control.

Those denials don't just waste time, they leave people unprotected. Weeks or months can pass while patients fight through appeals and paperwork. And the stakes are enormous: every gap in coverage increases the risk of an unintended pregnancy. Nearly half of all pregnancies in the United States already fall into that category.

For the millions insured through Medicaid, the picture is even more complicated. Patients may face quantity limits, mandatory generic substitution, or stricter prior authorization rules. Barriers that vary state by state. Two-thirds of women on Medicaid are in their reproductive years, yet their access to contraception often depends less on their medical needs than on their zip code.

For my patient and so many others, the message is clear: the system's rules matter more than your health, comfort, or choice. Every denial, every delay, every unnecessary hoop tells people the same thing, that their bodies don't get the final say. That's what makes the contraceptive coverage maze so devastating. It isn't just about insurance or paperwork. It's about control. And until we fix it, too many people will keep walking away from the pharmacy counter empty-handed, left to carry the cost of a system that was never built to put them first.

## When Belief Overrides Benefit: The Lasting Impact of *Burwell v. Hobby Lobby*

Your job shouldn't decide your birth control. Yet in 2014, *Burwell v. Hobby Lobby* gave certain for-profit companies exactly that power. It let an employer's beliefs dictate whether or not contraception was covered. The decision applied to "closely held" corporations, private companies owned and controlled by a small group of individuals, often family-run, but its ripple effects have reached far beyond that definition.

At the heart of the case was a law called the Religious Freedom Restoration Act, which protects people from laws that might interfere with their religious beliefs. The big question was whether a for-profit company could use that law to claim religious rights. The owners of Hobby Lobby, a Christian family, argued that they shouldn't have to include certain contraceptives in their employees' health insurance because those methods conflicted with their personal beliefs.

While the scientific consensus is that pregnancy begins at implantation, not fertilization, the owners' belief that certain contraceptives might prevent a fertilized egg from implanting and developing was central to their objection. That belief, rather than medical evidence, became the deciding factor in whether thousands of employees would be able to access federally mandated birth control through their insurance.

By siding with the company's belief over medical consensus, the Court set a precedent where healthcare coverage could be shaped by ideology rather than evidence-based standards. And because most Americans get their insurance through their employer, this isn't just about one company. The case created a framework where a single employer's objection could become a barrier for thousands of employees.

The concern extends beyond contraception. Under the same reasoning, other essential services, like infertility treatments, vaccinations, gender-affirming care, or mental health medications, could be excluded if they conflict with an employer's personal beliefs.

This isn't theoretical: it plays out in people's lives every day. If you're under 26 and still on your parent's insurance through a Catholic hospital, your birth control might not be covered at all. If you're a researcher working at a religiously affiliated university, fertility treatments like IVF may be excluded from your insurance coverage. If your employer objects to gender-affirming care or even certain common medications, your insurance may simply refuse to pay.

That leaves a fundamental question: how do we protect patients' access to consistent, evidence-driven care when the rules can shift based on who signs their paycheck?

## The Unequal Price of Choice

If contraceptive coverage with insurance is complicated, abortion access is even more restricted. It is structured in ways that often confuse, delay, and financially burden people who are trying to get care.

One of the biggest barriers is the Hyde Amendment. First passed in 1976, it bans federal Medicaid dollars from covering abortion except in rare cases: life endangerment, rape, or incest. On paper, it looks like a funding rule. In reality, it means that people who depend on Medicaid, low-income families, disabled people, young people, disproportionately people of color, are denied coverage for abortion, even though Medicaid covers almost every other kind of healthcare. More than 7.5 million women of reproductive age fall into this gap.

Critics sometimes say, "I don't want my tax dollars paying for abortion." But our tax dollars fund other reproductive healthcare, everything from prenatal care to labor and delivery, which is far more expensive than abortion. The government doesn't let individuals pick and choose which medical services their taxes support. Someone who doesn't believe in blood transfusions, chemotherapy, or dialysis doesn't get to block coverage for those services. Abortion is singled out as the exception, not because it isn't healthcare, but because of politics.

The Hyde Amendment doesn't save money, it creates inequality. People with private insurance can often use their coverage, while people on Medicaid, disproportionately low-income women and women of color, are denied that same right. The result is a two-tier system in which your ability to get care depends not on your medical needs, but on your income, your zip code, or your insurance card.

A handful of states have stepped in to cover abortion through Medicaid, but most have not. And wherever you live, the financial burden can be crushing. In states without Medicaid coverage, every dollar falls on the patient. For someone living paycheck to paycheck, that's not just expensive, it's impossible.

And because abortion is time sensitive, every barrier compounds the problem. Scraping together money, finding transportation, arranging time off—each delay pushes people further into pregnancy, making care harder to get and more costly. When Medicaid doesn't cover abortion, it doesn't just create a financial hurdle, it strips away real choice. People are left to continue pregnancies they had hoped to end, pregnancies they may not be ready to carry physically, financially, or emotionally.

For those already living at a financial disadvantage, this isn't just a healthcare barrier, it's an economic trap. It's often the same women who are already navigating poverty, unstable housing, or jobs without paid leave who are forced to have more children than they can afford. These are not the caricatured "welfare queens" of political talking points; they are real people making impossible choices in circumstances they didn't create. The economic impact of adding another child under those conditions can be devastating—stretching already thin resources, deepening poverty, and forcing families into cycles that are harder to break.

Even with private insurance, access isn't guaranteed. Many plans have high deductibles, meaning patients may still be responsible for the full cost. Some require prior authorizations or restrict coverage to specific clinical circumstances. Others limit abortion coverage to cases of medical emergency or sexual assault, creating additional administrative and emotional burdens for patients during already difficult moments. In some cases, insurers have required survivors of assault to file police reports or obtain physician attestations in order to qualify for coverage. No other form of healthcare requires patients to prove their trauma or justify their care in this way. It's invasive, retraumatizing, and a clear reminder that abortion is singled out for political reasons, not medical ones.

Geography now dictates who can and cannot get care. Since the US Supreme Court overturned *Roe v. Wade* in 2022, abortion access has fractured along state lines. Some states have banned or severely restricted it; others still protect it. The divide is stark: in the first half of 2023, nearly one in five abortion patients had to leave their home state for care. Double the share from just three years earlier.

For many, that means traveling hundreds or even thousands of miles, often with only days to plan. Patients juggle last-minute travel, unpaid time off, and childcare or eldercare—barriers that fall hardest on rural communities, hourly workers, and families already stretched thin. The result is a system in which medical need no longer sets the terms of care, your zip code does. Geography itself has become one of the biggest barriers to reproductive healthcare in America.

And while all of this happens on the ground, additional layers continue to unfold at the policy level. As this book was being written, Congress was actively negotiating whether to extend key Affordable Care Act subsidies that keep insurance premiums affordable for millions of people. In the middle of those negotiations came proposals to further restrict abortion coverage in private marketplace plans. The fact that coverage for abortion, already limited and segregated from federal funding, became a bargaining chip in those talks illustrates just how fragile access remains. Abortion coverage isn't stable policy; it's something that continues to be leveraged, traded, or tightened depending on the politics of the moment.

In practice, this has created a deeply unequal system. One where access to healthcare depends not only on medical need but also on insurance status, income, location, policy and personal circumstances. At its core, abortion is healthcare. And like any healthcare, it's only effective when it's timely, affordable, and accessible to the people who need it. When care is delayed or denied, the consequences extend far beyond the exam room, undermining health outcomes, economic stability, family well-being, and trust in the system itself.

## What Abortion Really Costs

Behind those structural barriers are staggering real-world costs. A medication abortion early in pregnancy typically ranges from $300 to $800. In-clinic procedures often start about $600 and can quickly rise into the thousands. And when people need care later in pregnancy, costs can soar into the tens of thousands. The longer someone is forced to wait, whether because of legal restrictions, trouble finding a provider, or time needed to raise money, the more complicated and expensive the care becomes. Fewer providers are willing or able to offer it, travel distances increase, and hospital-level interventions may be required. Each layer adds cost, and every dollar falls squarely on the patient.

In 2021, a friend and fellow advocate Kate Dineen had to travel 500 miles from Boston to Maryland after her son suffered a catastrophic stroke in utero. Even though Massachusetts had strong protections on paper, its 24-week cutoff meant she could not receive care at home. She and her husband were forced to pay more than $10,000 out of pocket for a feticidal injection. This is a standard step later in pregnancy that gently and painlessly stops the fetal heartbeat before a labor-induction abortion, ensuring the baby is delivered still and the procedure is safe and compassionate. It was just one step in the care she needed, yet it was legally out of reach in her own state and financially out of reach for so many families in the same position.

These are not abstract statistics; they are real families handed devastating bills in the middle of grief and crisis. When abortion isn't covered, the consequences reach far beyond the clinic visit. Families are driven into debt, forced to drain savings, or left without the option of care altogether. And because costs climb with every delay, the people already facing the greatest barriers—poverty, unstable housing, jobs without paid leave—are the ones penalized most harshly.

Denying coverage doesn't end abortion, but it reshapes who can access it, who must risk everything to obtain it, and who is left behind.

Kate shared with me:

> *"Abortion should never depend on your zip code or your bank account. No one should be forced to travel hundreds of miles and spend thousands of dollars just to get the care they need. Speaking out about my story isn't easy, but it's necessary—because silence only protects the system, not patients."*

Addressing these gaps isn't about politics. It's about ensuring that every person can make decisions about their own body, their own health, and their future—with dignity, compassion, and support.

## The Price of Asking for More

So here we are, in a system where what you need doesn't matter if it doesn't fit neatly into a reimbursement code. Where "covered" almost never means "enough." Where access depends less on medical need than on whether your insurance decides to recognize it. Where patients are punished for asking the wrong question at the wrong time, and providers are punished for daring to do more than the bare minimum.

Insurance isn't just a barrier, it's the architect of a system that delays, denies, and diminishes care. And it's easy to forget: you are more than a claim number. You're not a risk calculation or a line item on a quarterly report. You're a person who deserves care, real care, not just coverage.

So when they deny your prescription? Appeal it. When they refuse to cover the provider you need? Fight it. When they call something "not medically necessary," ask them exactly which medical degree taught them that.

The system is rigged. But it's not untouchable. And the first step to breaking it is refusing to play by rules written to make you lose.

# Chapter 6

# Broken System, Good People

*Not All Providers Are Bad, but They're Working in a System That Makes It Hard to be Good*

Most of us have at least heard of the Hippocratic Oath. That ancient promise physicians make to practice medicine ethically, to "do no harm," and to put the patient's well-being first. It's not just ceremonial language. Even though the exact wording has evolved over centuries, the core values, compassion, integrity, and service, still form the moral backbone of modern medical training.

And I believe most clinicians take that commitment seriously. They carry the weight of that oath with them into exam rooms, operating suites, and delivery wards. They enter medicine wanting to heal, to protect, to stand with their patients in some of life's most vulnerable and defining moments.

But good intentions, even paired with an oath, don't guarantee good outcomes, especially when the system itself works against them. Because while most OB-GYNs go into this field for the right reasons, they're practicing in a structure that makes it increasingly hard to live up to the ideals they swore to uphold.

It's easy to blame clinicians when patients feel dismissed, delayed, or harmed. Sometimes that blame is deserved. But more often, the reality is more complicated. Providers may want to do more, but policies limit their options. Hospital bylaws shaped by religious directives forbid them from offering contraception or abortion. Insurance companies deny coverage for treatments they know would help. State laws criminalize care they were trained to provide. Even the amount of time they spend with a patient can be dictated by billing codes, not medical judgment.

This chapter is about both sides of that equation: the providers who truly want to give better care and the policies that keep them from doing so. It's about people who entered medicine with good intentions and a system of rules, restrictions, and red tape that often makes it impossible for those intentions to translate into the care patients deserve.

## The Weight of the Work

OB-GYNs are burning out at alarming rates, in ways that affect both their lives and their patients'.

The pandemic accelerated a crisis that was already brewing. A national study found that by the end of 2021, more than 60% of US physicians reported burnout. Within obstetrics and gynecology, the numbers are even more sobering: one national survey of residents showed nearly two-thirds reported burnout, alongside overwhelming rates of anxiety, depression, and even suicidal thoughts. Another study in 2024 reported that 80% of OB-GYN trainees felt their mental health had been negatively affected by the pandemic. And among those burned out, almost half said they had experienced suicidal thoughts or knew someone who had.

This isn't just a "workplace issue." In reproductive healthcare, burnout becomes a patient issue. Every hour a provider spends fighting insurance denials or navigating endless clicks in an electronic health record is an hour taken away from actual patient care. And those clicks don't stop when the last patient leaves. Many OB-GYNs put in an extra one to two hours a day finishing charts after hours.

Burnout isn't only about stress. It's about erosion. Erosion of attention. Erosion of compassion. Erosion of the space and energy it takes to actually listen. When providers are stretched past their limits, visits get shorter, conversations get rushed, and symptoms slip through the cracks.

And patients feel it. We feel it in the hurried tone, the unanswered portal messages, the way we walk out of an appointment wondering, *Was that really it?*

This isn't about blaming doctors. It's about naming what's really happening: a system that pushes even good people past their breaking point, and leaves patients paying the price.

When burnout is this widespread, it's tempting to think the answer is just more self-care for clinicians, or maybe better scheduling. But the truth is, no amount of yoga classes or resilience training fixes a system where the barriers aren't just personal, they're structural. It's not only about exhausted providers; it's about the rules, directives, and policies that strip away their ability to act in the best interest of their patients.

Some of those constraints come from insurance companies and legislators. Others exist within the very institutions where care takes place. And few examples are more powerful, or more limiting, than Catholic hospitals.

## The Catholic Hospital Constraint: One in Seven Hospital Beds

Some OB-GYNs don't just fight the system, they work inside one that ties their hands. Catholic hospitals and other religiously affiliated health systems are governed not by medical standards, but by church directives. And their reach is enormous. Catholic health systems now control one in every seven hospital beds in the United States. And they're still expanding. As public and secular hospitals shrink, Catholic systems have surged. Of the nation's 10 largest health systems, 4 are Catholic, and together the 10 biggest now operate 394 short-term acute-care hospitals, a 50% jump in just two decades.

In some states, the presence is even more dominant. In Alaska, Iowa, South Dakota, Washington, and Wisconsin, 40% or more of hospital beds are in Catholic facilities. Which means that in many parts of the Midwest, the West, and especially in rural communities, the only hospital within reach may be Catholic-run.

And in those settings, what's evidence-based or patient-centered doesn't always matter. If the Ethical and Religious Directives for Catholic Health Care Services say no contraception, no sterilization, no abortion, then that's that. These rules prohibit entire categories of reproductive care. While some Catholic hospitals allow certain contraceptives, many restrict them, and sterilization is prohibited entirely. This matters because 98% of sexually active Catholic women have used contraception other than natural family planning, and more than half of women over 40 rely on sterilization. Services that, in many Catholic facilities, simply aren't available.

One of the clearest examples is postpartum sterilization, procedures performed right after childbirth to permanently prevent pregnancy, most often tubal ligation (known as getting your tubes tied) or bilateral salpingectomy (removing the fallopian tubes). For patients who are certain their families are complete, this is a safe, practical, one-and-done choice. It adds only a few minutes, doesn't change recovery, and spares the patient another surgery down the road. Nearly half of all sterilizations in the United States happen immediately after childbirth for this very reason. Lose that moment, and the barriers multiply: another surgery, another anesthesia, another recovery to plan for. And missing that window isn't just inconvenient, it can change someone's entire life.

But at Catholic hospitals, these procedures are off the table. The impact is measurable: women who deliver at Catholic hospitals have a 51% lower prevalence of postpartum sterilization compared to those delivering at non-Catholic hospitals, even after controlling for patient characteristics. Patients who are denied sterilization face a higher likelihood of unplanned *rapid repeat pregnancy*, getting pregnant again within 18 months. That short interval is linked to preeclampsia, preterm birth, and neonatal complications. In one chart review, nearly half (47%) of patients who were denied sterilization became pregnant within a year, double the rate of those who never asked.

And the restrictions don't stop with contraception or sterilization. They extend to abortion and miscarriage care, even when a patient's life is at risk. These directives have led to some of the most harrowing stories in reproductive medicine: patients experiencing life-threatening complications sent home untreated because the hospital refused to provide an abortion.

In 2024, Anna Nusslock, a physician herself, went to Providence St. Joseph Hospital in Humboldt County, California, after her water broke at just 15 weeks. She was bleeding heavily, carrying a pregnancy that could not survive, and told an abortion was necessary to protect her life and health. But because the hospital was bound by Catholic directives, doctors sent her home instead. With nothing but a bucket and towels. California law requires hospitals to provide emergency abortion care, yet Providence's religious policies overrode medical judgment and even state law. Dr. Nusslock is now suing, alongside the California Attorney General, to hold the hospital system accountable.

Her case is a reminder: these restrictions aren't limited to "red states" with abortion bans. They are happening in California, a state with some of the strongest reproductive protections in the country. They are happening in rural areas where Catholic hospitals may be the only option for miles. And they are happening to patients in the middle of emergencies, when delay or denial of care can mean the difference between life and death.

The takeaway is stark: where you deliver, or where you show up in crisis, can determine what care you're allowed to have. Not based on your health. Not based on your wishes. Not based on what's safest. But on religious rules you never agreed to. For millions of patients, that means the difference between ending childbearing on their own terms, or being forced into repeat surgeries, risky pregnancies, dangerous delays, and futures they didn't choose. And because Catholic health systems are growing while secular options shrink, this isn't just about one patient's story. It's a system-level constraint quietly reshaping what reproductive freedom looks like in this country. Even in places where the law says otherwise.

### *The Provider Workaround*

When hospital rules block care, many providers resort to what researchers call *workarounds*. Studies show how common this is: physicians coding procedures under alternative diagnoses to bypass Catholic directives. For example, recording an intrauterine device as treatment for heavy bleeding instead of contraception, or listing cancer prevention as the reason for removing fallopian tubes rather than sterilization. Interviews with OB-GYNs confirm the pattern. They describe the frustration of watching patients go through unnecessary second surgeries after a C-section because the hospital prohibited a tubal ligation, or relying on loopholes for sterilization that could disappear the moment hospital leadership decided to tighten policy.

But these workarounds come at a cost. Providers admit feeling "dishonest," forced to "purposely misdiagnose" patients, or ask "leading questions" just to fit care into an approved category. It leaves them trapped in a system where offering standard reproductive care means bending the truth. And the message patients receive is just as corrosive: that their needs aren't legitimate on their own. That reproductive healthcare has to be disguised, hidden, or justified as something else to be allowed at all.

## Post-Dobbs: The Criminalization of Medicine

Since the fall of *Roe v. Wade*, abortion has become not just a political issue, but a legal minefield for clinicians. In many states, laws now dictate what medical professionals can say, do, or offer. Care that was once considered standard practice is now grounds for criminal penalties. Physicians risk losing their licenses. Nurses and pharmacists face jail time. And every decision made in a clinic room, every conversation, every prescription, can be weaponized.

Across the country, dozens of states have enacted bans or near-total restrictions on abortion. Some cut off access as early as six weeks, long before many people even know they're pregnant. And here's the part that's often misunderstood: gestational age is calculated from the first day of your last menstrual period, not from the day you conceive or the day you miss your period. By that calculation, you're already about two weeks "pregnant" on the day you conceive.

That means a so-called six-week ban doesn't give you six full weeks to realize you're pregnant and make a decision. It gives you roughly two weeks from the point you know until the legal window closes. And that's only if your cycles are perfectly regular, you notice your missed period immediately, and you can get and afford a pregnancy test right away. If your cycles are irregular, it's easy to miss. If money is tight, you might wait before buying a test. If you're unsure, in denial, or hoping your period will come, the deadline can pass before you even realize it's open. Society often assumes people at the six-week mark have had that whole time to act, when in reality the clock started long before they even knew it was ticking.

These bans don't just affect abortion care, they've also muddied the waters about miscarriage management. Medically, the terminology for miscarriage overlaps with abortion. A spontaneous miscarriage is called a "spontaneous abortion" in medical records, and treatments like mifepristone and misoprostol or a surgical procedure called dilation and curettage are the same ones used for elective abortions. In states with strict bans, this creates dangerous gray zones. Many aren't even sure what's legal anymore, because the laws are intentionally vague, contradictory, punitive, and constantly changing or being challenged in court.

Providers are forced to consult legal teams before offering care. Pharmacies delay or deny medications. Hospitals hesitate to act until the patient is unstable enough to prove the pregnancy is no longer viable. These aren't theoretical risks. They're delays that have resulted in hemorrhage, infection, intensive care unit (ICU) admission, even death. And it's not a partisan issue. People across the political spectrum experience miscarriage and need abortion. But now, that care comes with legal scrutiny, unnecessary suffering, and lasting harm.

It's not just hypothetical. A recent qualitative study of 21 Wisconsin OB-GYNs practicing under a criminal abortion ban described exactly what it feels like to practice medicine when your license, livelihood, and freedom are on the line. Physicians reported "vague" and "uninterpretable" laws, hospital lawyers more concerned with protecting the institution than protecting patients, and constant uncertainty over what counted as "lifesaving" enough to justify care. Some described watching patients with pregnancy complications deteriorate—hemorrhage, become infected, even land in the ICU—because they weren't allowed to intervene until the danger was undeniable. Others talked about weighing whether to risk a felony conviction just to do what they knew was medically right. The result wasn't better medicine. It was substandard, delayed, fragmented care, and a generation of good clinicians forced into moral distress.

And the people paying the price are patients in crisis, trying to make urgent medical decisions in a system that's been rigged against them.

### Roe *Was Already a Compromise*

It's easy to imagine *Roe v. Wade* as a sweeping guarantee of abortion rights. But the truth is, *Roe* was never the ceiling, it was the floor. Decided in 1973, *Roe* did recognize a constitutional right to abortion. But it also gave states permission to limit abortion later in pregnancy, using the concept of "viability" as the dividing line. That was a compromise, and it meant that from day one abortion rights came with caveats.

Viability was never a clear medical standard. Even Justice Harry Blackmun, who wrote *Roe*, admitted the line was arbitrary. Doctors know that survival outside the womb depends on many factors: gestational age, fetal weight, genetics, and whether a neonatal intensive care unit is available. Even between 23 and 25 weeks, outcomes vary widely. Yet by tying rights to "viability," *Roe* downgraded the rights of pregnant people once they reached an uncertain and shifting medical threshold.

And while *Roe* stopped states from banning abortion outright, it left the door wide open for restrictions—and states rushed to walk through it. Mandatory waiting periods, parental involvement laws, mandatory ultrasounds, targeted clinic regulations, and the Hyde Amendment of 1976, which cut off Medicaid coverage of abortion, all chipped away at access. For millions, those barriers meant abortion was a right on paper but not always in practice.

That's why reproductive justice leaders began saying years ago that "*Roe* is the floor, not the ceiling." *Roe* set a minimum, it prevented the very worst bans, but it never guaranteed meaningful access. It left behind low-income patients, people of color, immigrants, minors, and anyone without the money or means to travel across state lines. It made abortion a right on paper, but not always in practice.

When *Dobbs* overturned *Roe*, it exposed and intensified the cracks that *Roe* never fixed. It has handed lawmakers and hospitals permission to treat patients as legal risks instead of human beings in need of care. And it has left both patients and clinicians navigating a system where medicine and law are at odds, and where the consequences of delay or denial are measured in blood loss, infection, and lives.

### The Clinical Impact: Delayed Care and Moral Distress

One of the most devastating consequences of post-*Dobbs* legislation has been the delay of essential care, not because providers don't know what to do, but because they're forced to wait until the situation becomes dire enough to justify action under the law.

Miscarriage care is one of the clearest, and most painful, examples. Miscarriage is far more common than most people realize: about 15–20% of known pregnancies end in miscarriage, and when you include very early losses before someone even knows they're pregnant, the number is closer to one in four. Many of these pregnancies are deeply wanted. Which means that when miscarriage happens, it's not just a medical event, it's often a profound and painful loss.

And the only thing more devastating than losing a pregnancy is being told by a compassionate, capable clinician, "I want to help you, but I legally can't... yet." In some states, the same medications and procedures used to treat miscarriage are also used for abortion, and providing them without meeting narrow legal criteria can mean massive fines, years in prison, the loss of a medical license, and devastating consequences for a provider's family. This isn't a one-time gamble, it's a risk they'd be asked to take again and again while also doing the basic work of their job, often in an environment policed by people with no medical training who are quick to place blame.

This isn't because clinicians stopped caring. It's because the system they're working in forces them to practice medicine with one hand tied behind their back. The same dynamic plays out in other emergencies: ectopic pregnancies left untreated while hospitals seek legal clearance, or cancer treatments postponed while providers weigh medical urgency against potential prosecution.

The ripple effect reaches even into counseling. In many states, the very language a clinician uses can be interpreted as a legal violation. That means patients aren't always given the full picture of their rights or options. Informed consent, the bedrock of ethical medicine, is compromised. Autonomy is stripped from people making some of the most difficult decisions of their lives, not because their doctor doesn't care, but because lawmakers have inserted themselves into the exam room.

And even when providers know their patient needs care they can't legally offer, referring them elsewhere can be a legal minefield. In some states, guiding a patient toward out-of-state abortion services could be considered aiding or abetting a crime. So instead of walking with patients through their care journey, clinicians are forced to step back and stay silent, knowing that silence can cost someone their health, or worse, their life.

## The Mental Health Toll on Providers

The psychological toll of these laws doesn't stop at the patient. Providers are suffering, too, and the impact is measurable. In a national study, 87% of OB-GYNs practicing under abortion bans reported anxiety about working in an unclear legal climate. Every clinical decision feels like a potential legal trap. Every conversation could be misinterpreted. Every moment in the exam room is shadowed by the fear of prosecution.

Symptoms of depression and anxiety are increasingly common in clinicians. Providers describe constant worry, difficulty sleeping, and the heavy weight of moral distress, knowing what their patients need, but being unable to deliver it. This isn't burnout in the traditional sense. It's a deep, ethical exhaustion that comes from being forced to choose between their oath and the law.

As one physician put it, "It used to be that any day you were going to work, you could get sued. And now, any day you go to work, you could be charged with a felony. And that additional anxiety just weighs on me."

## Legal Whiplash: What Georgia Shows Us

Georgia illustrates how rapidly shifting abortion laws destabilize medical practice and push providers into untenable conditions. This isn't just a state with an abortion ban, it's a case study in how legal uncertainty itself becomes a barrier to care.

In Georgia, the instability was immediate. After *Dobbs*, the state began enforcing a six-week abortion ban that dramatically restricted access. Then, in 2024, that ban was briefly overturned by a lower court, allowing care to resume temporarily. But within days, the Georgia Supreme Court reinstated the ban. Providers had to reopen services, call patients, and resume abortion care, only to stop again almost immediately. That kind of legal whiplash forces clinicians to pivot based on political shifts rather than medical evidence. It disrupts continuity of care, undermines clinical trust, and increases the risk of legal exposure with every change.

The signal to providers is clear: you cannot rely on the law to stay stable. Even when courts intervene, the infrastructure to deliver care has often already been dismantled, and the legal protections providers need can vanish overnight. This makes it nearly impossible to offer ethical, evidence-based reproductive healthcare, because every decision is shadowed by uncertainty.

## When the System Breaks: What Idaho Tells Us

In some states, abortion bans create uncertainty. In Idaho, they've created collapse. Idaho is no longer just unpredictable, it's what happens when extreme laws harden into daily reality. And the result is devastating.

Since the state's near-total abortion ban went into effect, providers have fled at a staggering pace. Just from 2022 to 2024, Idaho lost more than a third of its OB-GYNs, shrinking from 268 to 174, and over half of its maternal-fetal medicine specialists, the doctors who manage high-risk pregnancies. This exodus has left entire communities stripped of care. Over half of Idaho's 44 counties no longer have a single practicing OB-GYN.

The ripple effects are brutal. Labor and delivery units across the state have closed, forcing families to drive hours for something as basic as giving birth. The Idaho Hospital Association has even told patients to "establish a relationship with a doctor 100+ miles away," as if routine prenatal care, contractions, or hemorrhage can wait that long. In emergencies, women are stabilized locally and then transported more than 160 miles by ambulance, sometimes while actively miscarrying, sometimes while their babies are crowning.

Providers describe the impossible calculus of care under the ban. They're tasked to figure out "How much bleeding is too much? When can I step in without risking prosecution? What evidence would I need to defend myself in court?" Dr. Lauren Miller, a maternal-fetal medicine specialist who left for Colorado, voiced the fear driving so many out: "My greatest fear was being tried as a felon simply for saving someone's life." That fear is not unfounded. Idaho law threatens doctors with two to five years in prison and fines up to $20,000 for providing abortion care, even when the same procedures are lifesaving.

And for patients, the consequences are not abstract. What used to be a quick drive to the nearest hospital can now mean an hour or more on the road, sometimes while in active labor or experiencing an emergency. Families are left calculating the risks in real time: if a complication strikes, if bleeding starts, if a baby comes too quickly, those extra miles aren't just an inconvenience. They can be the difference between survival and loss.

This is what it looks like when the system breaks, not because providers stopped caring, but because the law made caring too dangerous to risk.

## When Bans Drive Doctors Out

Idaho isn't an outlier, it's a warning. Across the country, abortion bans are reshaping the OB-GYN workforce in ways that are quiet, steady, and devastating.

Future physicians are paying attention. After *Dobbs*, OB-GYN residency programs in states with abortion restrictions saw a 10.5% drop in applications. When surveyed, nearly 58% of third- and fourth-year medical students said they were "unlikely or very unlikely" to apply for residency in states with abortion restrictions. These aren't just career decisions. They're moral ones. Students are actively avoiding training in places where they'd be asked to abandon best practices or face legal risk for doing their jobs.

And for those already practicing, many are reaching a breaking point. Since *Dobbs*, 40% of OB-GYNs in abortion-ban states report feeling constrained in their ability to manage miscarriages and pregnancy-related medical emergencies. Not just abortion: miscarriage management, cancer treatment, contraception counseling. Routine care. Critical care. The kind of care they trained for, and are now barred from offering.

All of this is happening against a backdrop that was already strained. Even before *Dobbs*, the United States was projected to face a shortage of approximately 9,890 OB-GYNs by 2037. Now, that shortage is accelerating, especially in states where maternal health outcomes are already the worst in the nation.

We're seeing the consequences play out in real time. Wait times for routine exams and surgeries are growing. Labor and delivery units are closing. Rural care deserts are expanding. Emergency departments that once managed crises locally are now overwhelmed, with fewer specialists available to intervene early. In Idaho, where OB-GYNs have left in staggering numbers, maternal health outcomes have declined even further, placing the state in the bottom tier nationwide for pregnancy-related complications.

This isn't just about policy. It's about the slow collapse of a profession. Its about what happens to patients when the people trained to care for them are forced to leave, stay silent, or burn out. Providers aren't walking away because they've stopped caring. They're walking away because every option in front of them is untenable.

Stay, and they risk arrest or professional ruin. Stay, and they may have to compromise the care they know is right just to protect themselves legally. But leaving isn't an easy answer either. It means abandoning the patients who trust them, often in communities where no one else is left. It means deepening the very crisis they've spent their careers trying to solve.

There is no good option. And that's the point. These laws are designed to create no-win scenarios, punishing clinicians for doing what they were trained to do, and forcing the people who still want to help into silence, hesitation, or exile.

### New Pathways to Care

Recent data makes one thing abundantly clear: abortion didn't vanish after *Dobbs*, it was rerouted. According to the WeCount national study, by mid-2024 nearly 98,000 abortions were happening every month across the United States. That's slightly higher than the immediate post-*Dobbs* period, not because the need suddenly grew, but because patients and clinicians found new ways to meet it when old pathways closed. Roughly one in five abortions were completed through telehealth, up from just 4% in early 2022. And nearly 9,700 abortions each month were provided under new state "shield laws," where clinicians in protective states legally prescribe across state lines to patients in banned or restricted states.

The state-level data tell the same story. In Texas, despite a total ban, roughly 2,800 residents each month still obtained abortion pills through telehealth from shield-law states. Louisiana and Mississippi averaged around 600 and 390 telehealth abortions per month, respectively. The care didn't disappear; the burden simply shifted.

This is what a two-tiered system looks like. In supportive states, patients receive local, timely care. In banned or highly restricted states, patients are pushed into legal gray zones, long drives, and online care networks. Telehealth and shield-law models have become lifelines, but they shouldn't have to be. They exist because lawmakers forced medicine to contort around politics.

Researchers caution that even these numbers undercount reality. They don't fully capture self-managed care or non-clinician support routes. Which means the real scale of adaptation, and the emotional and logistical strain it places on both patients and providers, is likely much higher.

If there's anything hopeful here, it's that care didn't vanish. It evolved through the people who refused to look away. The WeCount data isn't just a record of what's happening; they're a record of who kept showing up when it mattered most. It shouldn't take this much courage to provide standard medical care, but right now, it does. And these numbers are proof that good people are still doing the work, even when the system has stopped making it possible.

## What This Means for You

Across every level of this system, from overworked residents to physicians silenced by hospital policy to clinicians risking prosecution just to do their jobs, the same truth repeats: most people in medicine are still trying to do the right thing inside a structure that keeps making it harder to. The burnout, the Catholic hospital restrictions, the criminalization of care, the scramble to build telehealth and shield-law networks, they're all different symptoms of the same disease: a healthcare system that prioritizes politics, profit, and self-preservation over patient well-being.

And yet, in every corner of it, there are people still showing up. The doctors who rewrite policies to fit patient needs. The nurses who quietly advocate for care their hospitals won't approve. The clinicians who stay on call, not because it's safe, but because they can't stomach walking away. Care continues because people—providers, advocates, patients—keep pushing it forward.

That's the story beneath all the statistics and headlines. Not a system that's working, but a workforce trying to save it from collapse. Not a loss of compassion, but a shortage of conditions that enable it to thrive.

So where does this leave you, and what does it mean for your care?

It means the provider who seems rushed may not necessarily be dismissive, they might be seeing 30 patients today because half their colleagues left. It means the one who can't answer your questions about contraception might be working at a Catholic hospital where policy supersedes medicine. It means the person who seems burned out might be spending hours each evening fighting insurance denials instead of going home to their family.

None of this excuses poor care. You still deserve compassion, time, and answers. But understanding the forces at play changes how you can respond. Both things can be true: you can be dismissed, gaslit, or harmed by a clinician—and it can also be true that they're working inside a system that grinds down even the best intentions. Holding that complexity doesn't mean giving anyone a pass; it just means seeing the full picture.

Instead of wondering "What's wrong with me?" when care feels cold or rushed, you can ask, "What's wrong with this system?" Instead of blaming yourself for a bad experience, you can recognize when you're witnessing systemic failure in real time.

This knowledge becomes your armor. When a provider doesn't have time for your questions, you know it's not because your questions don't matter, it's because the system doesn't value the time it takes to answer them. When your pain gets dismissed, you know it's not because you're imagining it. It's because the system wasn't designed to take it seriously.

The providers who are fighting to stay, fighting to do better within these constraints? They need patients who understand what they're up against. And the system that's failing you both? It needs people who refuse to accept that this is just "how healthcare works."

Because it doesn't have to be. And the first step toward change is refusing to pretend it's fine.

# Chapter 7

# The Trauma We Carry In

*When the System Doesn't See Trauma, It Risks Creating More of It*

We don't talk about the things that break us. Most of us don't want to, if we're honest.

We don't talk about the assault. The miscarriage. The diagnosis that changed everything. The birth that left you bleeding and alone.

We don't talk about the memories we'd rather forget, or the ones we've shoved down again and again. And society makes it easy to keep them buried. There's no safe place to unpack them, no steady hand to help release the pressure before it builds. So the trauma sits there, like a pressure cooker, heat rising, steam trapped beneath the surface.

And it doesn't just stay buried inside you. Trauma shows up in the exam room. It shapes how your body reacts to procedures, what symptoms you report (or don't), the diagnoses you're given, and the way you're treated. What lives unspoken in your past can change how care unfolds in the present.

Sometimes that pressure escapes in quiet, almost invisible ways. A fleeting flashback. A voice in your head you thought you'd silenced. A sudden feeling in your body you can't name. Small reminders that the lid was never really sealed, that the past is still there, waiting for its moment to break through.

Other times, the release is sudden and all-consuming. The lid blows open, and everything rushes out at once. Maybe it's the insertion of a speculum. An ultrasound probe with an image flashed on the screen. A provider's hand resting on your knee when you weren't expecting it. And suddenly, what you've held down for years is right there again. Loud, sharp, impossible to ignore.

This is the part we rarely name: how lonely it is to carry all of that in silence. How isolating it feels to walk through the world like everyone else is fine, wondering if you're the only one who can't seem to just "get over it."

You're not the only one. Far from it.

Trauma isn't just the "big" things people name: assault, catastrophic loss, war. It's also the repeated harms and violations that accumulate over time: the doctor who dismissed your pain, the partner who controlled your choices, the job that broke you down, the birth that wasn't what you were promised. Trauma is anything that overwhelms your ability to cope and leaves a mark. On your mind, your body, or the way you move through the world. Some of it is visible. Most of it isn't. All of it matters.

And the truth is, trauma doesn't vanish because we aren't talking about it, or because no one asks in the first place. It lives in the body. It shapes how we move through care. A routine Pap smear can feel like a violation. A transvaginal ultrasound can summon memories you thought you'd locked away. And when no one asks, it confirms the worst fear: that your pain doesn't matter here. Worse, the shame culture around anything tied to women's bodies tells you it must be your fault anyway. That if you can't handle it, you're weak, dramatic, or broken. So you push it aside, force a smile, and try to act like you're fine.

Some patients flinch. Others go numb. Some cancel appointments, ghost follow-ups, or grit their teeth through procedures they don't fully understand. Providers, often rushed, rarely trained in trauma-informed care, miss the signs, or mistake them for "difficult," "noncompliant," or "anxious."

## The Prevalence We Don't Acknowledge

Trauma isn't rare. It's nearly universal, especially for women in healthcare settings. In one study of urban women seeking care, 86% reported at least one traumatic event in their lifetime, and many experienced more than one. For a significant share, those events left lasting scars: nearly one in three had experienced post-traumatic stress disorder (PTSD) at some point, and more than half of those with PTSD also lived with depression. These aren't abstract statistics—they're daily realities. If trauma hasn't touched you directly, the odds are overwhelming that it has touched your best friend, your sister, your mother. Trauma is woven into the fabric of women's lives, whether or not it's spoken aloud.

Here's the hard truth: sexual violence is far more common than most of us want to admit. By conservative estimates, nearly one in five women in the United States has been raped. And if you widen the lens to harassment, unwanted touching, groping, intimidation, sexual comments, the number is staggering. More than 80% of women have experienced harassment, assault, or both.

The reality is this: there is no lesser or greater version of harm. Whether it's force, pressure, or intimidation, the body remembers. And it is all violence. If any of this includes you, your experience is real. It matters. And you deserve care and safety.

And it almost never looks like the "stranger in the alleyway" we've been taught to fear. More than half of women who survive rape say the perpetrator was an intimate partner. Another 40% say it was someone they knew: an acquaintance, a friend, someone they trusted enough to let in.

For many, the violence began unbearably young. Nearly half were still children the first time it happened, and four out of five weren't yet 25.

Then there's another kind of trauma we rarely name out loud: medical trauma. It's not just a "bad experience" at the doctor's office. It's the harm that lingers in the body and the mind, reshaping how safe, or unsafe, healthcare feels. It can come from being ignored while bleeding, from having a procedure done without true consent, from being shamed instead of supported, or from having your pain written off as exaggeration. These aren't inconveniences; they're violations that stick, long after the appointment ends.

And medical trauma collides with identity, history, and bias. For Black, Indigenous, and other patients of color, racial trauma overlays every medical encounter: pain dismissed, symptoms ignored, dignity questioned. For LGBTQ+ patients, it can show up in being misgendered, erased from intake forms, or denied gender-affirming care. For people with disabilities, it's providers speaking to caregivers instead of to them, assuming incompetence, or treating their body as a problem to be fixed instead of a life to be lived. For survivors of sexual violence, the setting itself—a gown, stirrups, a stranger's hands—can bring old terror rushing back.

Then there are the kinds of trauma that rarely make it onto an intake form. Living with an eating disorder or disordered eating. Growing up in an unsafe home. Living with a parent who struggled with addiction. Enduring neglect. Watching violence unfold around you. Living in poverty, carrying the constant stress of financial instability, or navigating the fear and uncertainty of immigration status. Facing discrimination, racism, or social rejection that chips away at your sense of safety.

These experiences are all traumas that live in the body and often collide with medical care. Yet they often remain unnamed in a chart, and echo back in the exam room, especially when someone is returned to a position of powerlessness. These traumas all shape how people show up in medical care, even if the system may not ask about them.

Every one of us walks into care carrying our own history, whether or not anyone else can see it. Some of it is written on our bodies, some of it lives quietly in memory, but all of it matters. Trauma takes many forms, but it always comes back to power and the ways it's taken away. And in healthcare, where you can't simply walk out when things go wrong, the stakes are even higher.

Those scars, whether born of sexual violence, racism, sexism, homophobia, fat-shaming, ableism, medical neglect, or something else entirely, shape how we trust, how we heal, and how we're treated. Even if they've never been named, even if no one else recognizes them, they are real. And they deserve care that honors them. Because if we can't name them, we can't change them.

And here's what honoring them should look like when you walk into care: You should be asked for consent before someone touches your body—not just once, but throughout the visit. You should be told what's about to happen, in plain language, with a chance to ask questions. You should feel like your words matter. If you say you're in pain, scared, or uncomfortable, that should shape what happens next. You should never feel punished for needing an extra pause, a support person in the room, or a different approach.

Good care doesn't erase trauma, but it doesn't add to it. At its best, it helps you feel safer than you did when you walked in. That's the baseline you deserve. And if you don't get it, that's not a personal failing, it's a system failing. Knowing that difference is the first step toward protecting yourself inside it.

## When Birth Itself Becomes the Trauma

Birth is supposed to be a threshold moment. A crossing into parenthood, a memory that stays for life. For some, it is just that: challenging, exhausting, but ultimately joyful. For others, it becomes something very different. What should be an act of care turns into trauma.

The risks aren't just from medical emergencies like hemorrhage or emergency surgery; they include feeling powerless, not being listened to, being left alone when you're scared, or having procedures done without consent. Depression during pregnancy, fear of childbirth, and poor overall health all raise the risk of trauma, but so do preventable system failures: fragmented care, provider burnout, and a model that treats emotional safety as optional instead of essential.

In childbirth alone, one in three people describe their birth as traumatic, 17% of birthing people experience symptoms of PTSD, and about 4% of women go on to develop full PTSD from the birth. With 3.6 million births in the United States in 2024, that translates to roughly 145,000 new cases of birth-related PTSD each year.

And these aren't just "bad memories." PTSD after medical or reproductive trauma can mean flashbacks, panic attacks, nightmares, avoiding care, and intense anxiety about future pregnancies. It's why some people delay or avoid having more children. Not because they don't want them, but because the thought of another birth feels unbearable.

If this has been your experience, you are not alone. Your story is real. And the failure is not yours.

## Birth Doesn't Have to Be Blissful

When I got engaged, everyone told me I'd cry when I found the right wedding dress. That I'd just know. That there would be this magical, aha moment. So I waited for it. I tried on over 100 dresses, and it never came. Eventually, I had to accept that for me, there wasn't going to be a lightning bolt dress moment. That experience wasn't universal, no matter how much people swore it would be.

We do the same thing with pregnancy and birth. We assume people will be glowing, thrilled, elated. The first thing most people say after a pregnancy announcement is "Congratulations!"

As if there's only one script to follow. No pause to acknowledge that it might not feel like a fairytale at all.

I was recently talking with my best friend, whose first delivery was traumatic, and she was weighing her options for future fertility and delivery. She had prepared so carefully for her first birth. Took all the hypnobirthing classes, hired a doula, planned for it to be peaceful and empowering. Instead, after three days of failed induction, she ended up with preeclampsia, an unplanned C-section, and her newborn was in the neonatal intensive care unit (NICU) for a week.

It was one of the hardest times of her life. For her, the next birth carries the weight of hope and redemption. The goal that maybe this time she'll finally get that aha moment. And it hit me: this was the wedding dress all over again, only on a much more profound scale. We're told to expect transcendence, to wait for magic. But what if it doesn't come? What if labor and delivery just . . . suck?

Here's the truth: it's okay if birth wasn't the best day of your life. It doesn't mean you failed. It doesn't mean you don't love your kids or love being a parent. Sometimes birth isn't blissful or empowering. Sometimes it's just the day your baby was born. And that's enough.

And still, there's more space here than we're usually given. For some, birth is profoundly healing or transformative. For others, it is deeply traumatic. And for many, it lives somewhere in between. A day that was hard, complicated, or simply "fine," without needing to be cast as either magical or horrifying. Part of why it's so hard to hold these possibilities is because we're rarely shown them. Media usually offers only two scripts: the screaming woman barely surviving or the glowing mother basking in bliss. Family stories are limited, too: you might only know your mother's version, or hear a single story from an aunt, without realizing how different each birth can be. And in many communities, the nuances—the ambivalence, the ordinary, the messy middle—are never spoken aloud at all.

That silence does more than leave us unprepared. It narrows what feels possible. If all you've ever heard is that birth is either magical or miserable, where do you put your own complicated reality? If your experience doesn't fit the script, you can end up questioning yourself instead of questioning the system that made room for only two narratives.

The truth is, birth doesn't have to be only one thing. It can be awful and beautiful, mundane and profound, disappointing and miraculous—all at once. Making space for that complexity doesn't diminish anyone's story. It honors them. And it gives us all more room to breathe. And yet, even with all this complexity, most of us don't get to hear about it until we're already in the thick of it.

Before someone joins the birthing club, we rarely speak honestly about what it's like. But once your belly is big enough, suddenly everyone feels entitled to share their story. I remember being a week away from my first delivery when the checkout woman at the grocery store launched into the details of her own birth. I wanted to scream—not now, not like this.

That's the contradiction: we desperately need more space to talk about birth, but not through unsolicited stories that land on an unprepared stranger. There's a difference between creating safe, intentional conversations and trauma dumping on someone just because they happen to look pregnant. The same way we talk about consent in other parts of life, we need a kind of narrative consent here, too: "Can I share my experience with you?" goes a long way toward making a story feel supportive instead of overwhelming.

And then I've spoken to so many people after their first birth where so much seems to hinge on the "success" of a second birth. The redemption, if you will. If the first didn't go as planned—if there was an unplanned C-section, a hemorrhage, a baby in the NICU, or even just a sense of being silenced or dismissed—then the next pregnancy often carries the weight of rewriting that story. Suddenly, it's not just about welcoming another child. It's about redemption, repair, a second chance at the story you thought you'd get the first time.

The catch is, most of the time people haven't truly healed from the first birth by the time they're entering the second. They carry unresolved grief, fear, or anger into the delivery room, hoping the next experience will wipe the slate clean. But trauma doesn't vanish just because another baby is on the way. When it goes unacknowledged, the pressure builds: to make the next birth "perfect," to finally achieve the elusive experience you were promised. And if the second birth doesn't deliver that neat redemption arc, the disappointment can feel even heavier.

Birth defies categories—it's rarely all bliss or all pain, and most often lives somewhere in the complicated middle. You can plan for months, make every choice carefully, and still find the day unfolding in ways you never expected. Sometimes it's beautiful and hard at the same time. Sometimes it feels ordinary when you hoped for extraordinary. Sometimes it's all of those things layered together.

What matters most isn't whether your story matched the script you were handed, but whether you felt seen in it. And if you didn't—if your birth was traumatic, silencing, or left you carrying more pain than joy—that doesn't make your story any less real. It means it's yours to hold, to process, to grieve, and to move through in your own time. Birth doesn't stop shaping us the moment the baby arrives. It lingers, it echoes, and sometimes it demands healing.

However it unfolded—joyful, complicated, traumatic, or somewhere in between—it is yours. And while "yours" might not feel like enough right now, it's also the starting point. The place from which healing, support, and new meaning can grow.

## The Silence That Protects Us—And Hurts Us

Only 7.6% of trauma survivors share their history with a gynecologist. And there's a reason so many people stay silent. Sometimes we want to forget. Sometimes we just want to make it through the appointment without falling apart. I get it. I've done it. As a survivor of childhood sexual abuse, I've filled out intake forms and left that question blank. I've said "no history" when I didn't want to explain. Even with all my clinical training, even knowing what I know, I couldn't always find the words when a provider assumed there was nothing to speak of. Because sometimes, saying it out loud just doesn't feel worth the cost.

What I didn't understand then—but is painfully clear to me now, both personally and professionally—is that trauma doesn't stay in the past just because we don't name it. It shows up in the body, in our mental health, in the ways we move through care.

The research confirms what many of us have felt in our bones: having a trauma history puts you at significantly higher risk for anxiety and depression at baseline, and even more so in the postpartum period.

When I was pregnant with my first child, I wanted so desperately for it to be a girl. I couldn't wait to raise a powerful woman. It was October 2017. I walked out of the ultrasound room having just confirmed it was a boy, looked down at my phone, and saw the first public accusations against Harvey Weinstein. Men. Always men. Boys. A son. How could it be? My blood boiled.

As woman after woman came forward with her own #MeToo story, it was like a dam breaking. Except I wasn't ready for the flood. Every headline, every post, every whispered conversation felt like another shove into memories I had fought to keep buried. The trauma didn't just resurface; it forced its way out, uninvited, dragging me with it. There was no pause button. No way to set it aside while I figured out how to breathe again.

And all of this was happening inside a body already stretched to its limit. I was nauseous and exhausted, with a boy growing inside me. A boy I hadn't expected, at a moment when men's violence against women was all anyone was talking about and all I could feel. I couldn't escape the reminder that I was carrying the future while the past was pounding at the door, demanding to be let in.

It wasn't some cathartic release. It was agonizing. Confusing. Miserable. I had no control over it. And it triggered me. Because for another time, I felt like I was being held captive by trauma I never agreed to carry.

After my son was born, I couldn't handle even the simplest things without being jolted back into my past trauma. Breastfeeding was miserable. It hurt. I didn't know what the hell I was doing, and my son wouldn't latch. That's a common experience for many new parents, especially first-time ones. But the memory of I forcing his head toward my breast as he wailed, being struck by the unbearable feeling that neither of us had consented to this, will always be burned into my mind. It was beyond triggering. Then came the nightmares. Then the flashbacks. I slipped into intense postpartum anxiety and depression.

I had *everything*. The medical training. The resources. The support system. If anyone should've seen it coming, it was me. And then, like so many victims, I blamed myself. I told myself I should've been tougher, more prepared. I was an OB-GYN PA, for crying out loud. How could I be falling apart?

The same words echoed in my head that have played for decades. "What's wrong with me?" and "I'm broken."

But the truth is and what I wish I could have told myself is that it wasn't my fault. None of it was my fault.

And as it related to the worsening postpartum anxiety and depression, no one screened me. No one prepared me. No one connected the dots between my past and what might surface after birth because no one even knew about my past. No one had ever asked the tough questions nor did I ever feel brave or vulnerable enough to be able to share.

If someone, anyone, had asked me about history of trauma, my red flags would've lit up like a Christmas tree. But no one did. And I fell through the cracks of a system I thought I could trust. I'm a clinician, but in this instance, I was a patient. And as a patient, I still slipped through. Even with my training. Even having been on the inside.

And my story isn't rare. It's just rarely told.

## When Trauma Flares Up

For many survivors, the doctor's office isn't just a place for care. It's a place where trauma echoes, quietly, or not so quietly, through every part of the experience.

For survivors of sexual violence, medical care can be its own battlefield. A routine gynecologic exam isn't routine at all when it pulls you back into memories you've fought to leave behind. Studies show that about half of survivors experience flashbacks or heightened anxiety during genital exams. And the numbers only tell part of the story. Survivors describe sitting on that table and feeling their body betray them: panic rising, memories rushing in, emotions flooding so fast they can't catch their breath. Some feel intrusive thoughts they can't quiet, some relive the trauma through "body memories," and some disconnect entirely. Watching it happen as though to someone else.

For patients with current or past eating disorders, the exam room can be its own minefield. Triggers show up everywhere: stepping on a scale, hearing body commentary during an exam, following fasting instructions, or receiving a care plan that hinges on weight instead of symptoms. None of that is small. Each one is an opportunity to center safety.

Infertility and pregnancy loss also carry their own weight. Grief that lives in the body and can erupt with the simplest prompt: a baby crying in the next room or a provider's question about "family planning." Like other forms of trauma, these aren't side stories. They shape how patients enter care, how they experience it, and what it takes to feel safe inside it.

The truth is, the triggers are everywhere. It might be the simple act of being touched, even somewhere neutral. It might be the power dynamic of lying back while someone else makes decisions. It might be the removal of clothing, or the way an exam zeroes in on pain, on brokenness. And it's not just pelvic exams. Colonoscopies, endoscopies, any procedure that involves instruments entering the body can echo the violence of sexual trauma closely enough to unleash a posttraumatic reaction. What the medical system sees as "standard care" can feel like reopening the wound.

And yet, trauma is still treated like the exception. Most providers get little to no training in how to recognize it, let alone how to respond in ways that prevent more harm. If a patient tenses up or pulls away, it's rarely met with the curiosity or care that moment calls for. If they ask for a pause, it might be met with an eye roll. If they cancel altogether, no one asks why. And the real reason is lost, never followed up on.

But trauma doesn't make you a bad patient. It means you've been through something that changed how your body experiences the world. That doesn't deserve judgment, it deserves care.

## Your Body Remembers

And the biology backs that up. Survivors of sexual violence don't just carry emotional scars, their bodies actually change. Research shows that trauma can disrupt the hypothalamic-pituitary-adrenal axis, the body's central stress response system. In simpler terms, trauma can rewire the way your body handles stress, leaving the "alarm system" stuck on high alert. That overdrive shows up in both the brain and the body as the hallmark symptoms of PTSD: flashbacks, hypervigilance, and exhaustion.

Researchers argued that treating PTSD without acknowledging its biological, psychological, and social roots is not only ineffective, it's negligent. Medication alone won't work if the mind is still carrying unprocessed fear. Therapy alone won't stick if the body's stress hormones are still out of balance. And neither will be enough if a survivor is left in a community that doubts or blames them. In other words: trauma isn't just in your head. It's in your nervous system. It's in your hormones. It's in your cells.

Trauma leaves fingerprints everywhere. The combat veteran who can't sit with his back to the door in a restaurant. The assault survivor whose jaw aches every time she hears footsteps behind her. The patient who bursts into tears during a routine blood draw because the smell of antiseptic jolts her back to a hospital bed she never wanted to be in. These aren't overreactions. They're the body remembering, and bracing for, what it's been through.

And here's the devastating part: we have known this for decades. We've had the research. We've had the science. For a long time. And yet trauma-informed care still isn't the standard. Survivors are still being retraumatized in medical settings every single day.

## Building Safer Exams

The system can do better, and we know trauma-informed care works. Research from the Veterans Health Administration found that when clinics implemented trauma-informed approaches, patient anxiety dropped by 43% and satisfaction rose by 31%. Those numbers prove what survivors already know in their bones: when care feels safe, healing is possible.

That kind of safety begins before the exam even starts. A trauma-informed provider will take time to build trust while you're still clothed, ask about your history, and check in on what would help you feel comfortable. You have the right to say what you need, whether that's a slower pace, more explanation, or choosing who's in the room. You're not alone. Research shows that up to 35% of gynecologic exams trigger trauma responses. So these small shifts aren't extras; they're what make the difference between care that retraumatizes and care that respects.

During the exam itself, you can ask for options. Some patients prefer to insert the speculum themselves. Others want the provider to narrate each step out loud so nothing comes as a surprise. You can ask to skip stirrups if possible, or request that exposure time be kept to a minimum. These may sound like small details, but they can make the difference between feeling retraumatized and feeling respected.

The research backs it up: patients who self-insert the speculum report significantly lower anxiety and discomfort. Vaginal self-swabs for sexually transmitted infection testing are essentially on par with clinician-collected cervical swabs—catching about the same number of infections (92% versus about 95% sensitivity) and ruling them out just as reliably (98% versus about 99% specificity). These tools give patients more autonomy, especially survivors.

When we don't make room for trauma, the fallout is real: panic attacks, dissociation, avoidance. Sometimes people stop coming altogether. Conditions worsen. Diagnoses get delayed. Trust breaks down. Not just in one provider, but in the entire system. And the ripple effects are expensive. Survivors use more healthcare, rack up more costs, and are more likely to end up in emergency rooms when things finally spiral.

## Consent-Based Care Still Isn't the Standard

Trauma-informed care is about respecting what someone says they need. But the reality is, it isn't the standard. And it's not surprising—OB-GYNs receive little to no training on how to care for patients through that lens. The gap is staggering: only 20% of OB-GYN programs provide annual trauma-informed care training, and more than a quarter offer no trauma curriculum at all. Among those currently in training, just one in four residents say they are satisfied with how they're being taught to address interpersonal trauma.

Even today, consent-based care is too often treated like a courtesy instead of a requirement. Part of the reason is time. It's quicker not to ask, not to pause, not to explain. But the deeper truth is that medical training never built it in.

When I perform pelvic exams, I try to rebuild that trust from the start. I ask simple, explicit questions: "Would you like me to ask for consent before each step? Would you prefer I explain what I'm doing as we go, or only flag moments you might feel discomfort? Or would you rather silence, with the option to speak up if something feels off?" These aren't complicated asks. They're human ones.

And yet, it wasn't until 2024 that federal guidance finally required written consent for pelvic, breast, prostate, or rectal exams performed under anesthesia in teaching hospitals. Think about that: until very recently, patients were still being used for "practice" without their knowledge.

I know, because I was once asked to do it. Back in 2014, I was a physician associate (PA) student, I was eager to follow orders and a supervising doctor turned to me during a surgery and asked if I wanted to practice a pelvic exam on the anesthetized patient, because "it's the perfect time to learn since everything is relaxed." I froze. Not because I didn't know what felt right, but because I wasn't sure if I had the power to say no. Would pushing back risk my standing in the rotation? My evaluations? My future in the program? Before I could even respond, a nurse in the operating room stepped in and shut it down. I was relieved, but that moment has never left me. That split-second tension, between what your gut tells you is wrong and what the hierarchy seems to demand, is exactly what the research describes.

In a multi-institutional survey, nearly three-quarters of students said pelvic exams under anesthesia should only be performed with explicit informed consent. But the data also revealed something deeper: first-year students were more likely to call nonconsensual exams unethical than upper-year students. As students advanced through training, their outrage dulled. The longer they spent in clinics and operating rooms, the more they absorbed the unspoken message that this was "just how it's done."

That quiet shift is called *ethical erosion*: the process where fresh eyes and gut instincts give way to the normalization of practices that once felt clearly wrong. It doesn't mean students stop caring. It means the culture of medicine, with its hierarchies and hidden curriculum, teaches them to override their own discomfort. Many reported moral distress—knowing something felt wrong, but feeling pressure to comply with expectations from supervising physicians.

And the truth is, this isn't just about pelvic exams under anesthesia. It's a window into medicine as a whole. What those surveys show—that students enter training with clear ethical instincts and leave more willing to accept questionable practices—reflects the same pattern I've seen again and again. The longer you're immersed in the system, the easier it becomes to stop questioning it.

Some might say I don't have the credentials to write this book, or that I shouldn't critique residency at all. After all, I never went through it myself. I'm not a Doctor. But the ethical erosion that happens during residency is my counter to that argument. The lack of critical criticism of the whole system. It's … precisely because I didn't train inside of it, I wasn't pulled into its gravity. I wasn't conditioned to accept its blind spots as "just the way things are."

Instead, I got to stand at the edge of the system, close enough to understand it, but with enough distance to see it clearly. And from that vantage point, I kept noticing things that others around me didn't. Practices that had become so routine that no one blinked, while I kept thinking, *Is this really the best the system can do?* Again and again, the answer was no. But when you're steeped in a culture that rewards compliance, speed, and silence, it gets harder to see those cracks.

That's why ethical erosion matters. It's not just about pelvic exams under anesthesia, it's about medicine itself. The longer you're immersed, the easier it is to override your own instincts and stop asking the uncomfortable questions. My position outside of residency meant I kept asking them. And if this book does anything, I hope it gives others permission to do the same.

## When #MeToo Came for Medicine

The cultural wave of #MeToo didn't stop at film sets or corporate boardrooms. It crashed into medicine, too. For decades, women were never encouraged to talk about it. The trauma, the pelvic exam that left them shaking, the ultrasound that brought back memories they thought were buried, the provider who didn't stop when they said "that hurts." The culture didn't give us language for those experiences, and medicine certainly didn't invite us to name them.

Then #MeToo ripped the silence wide open. Stories poured out, not just about workplaces and boardrooms but about clinics and delivery rooms. And for a moment, there was validation. A reckoning that we were not alone. Women could finally say, *This happened to me too.* And instead of being dismissed, they were met with a chorus of recognition. The pain that had been carried quietly for so long was suddenly visible, and undeniable.

For many, the trauma had begun long before they entered a clinic. Survivors of sexual assault, abuse, or violence walked into healthcare already carrying scars. A speculum, stirrups, or the loss of control that comes with lying on an exam table could rip those wounds wide open. For others, the trauma was born inside the healthcare system itself. They weren't retraumatized, they were traumatized by medicine. By procedures done without true consent. By a provider who ignored a plea to stop. By systems that lacked even the most basic safeguards.

The conviction of Larry Nassar made this reality impossible to ignore. Here was a physician who, under the guise of medical care, assaulted hundreds of young athletes over years. Protected by institutions that failed to listen to survivors and failed to enforce guardrails that should have kept them safe. Nassar's case was an extreme, but it was not an aberration. It revealed the devastating cost of silence, the absence of oversight, and the way medicine can be weaponized against those it's meant to protect. Poor guidelines, weak accountability, and a culture that prioritized reputation over safety left thousands of women vulnerable.

In the wake of this reckoning, the language of "trauma-informed care" crossed over from social work into the mainstream of medicine. Suddenly it wasn't just activists and survivors using the term, it was appearing on medical conference agendas, in training sessions, in hospitals eager to show they were listening. But here's the truth: these changes didn't come from the top down. They weren't mandated by medical schools or governing boards. They rose up from the grassroots. Patients demanding better, survivors refusing to stay silent, culture forcing the profession to catch up.

And the evidence backs this push. Systematic reviews show that trauma-informed practices in healthcare—staff education, clinic redesigns, and policy shifts—can improve patient well-being and reduce retraumatization. Even short trainings have been shown to boost clinicians' ability to recognize and respond to trauma. The American Medical Association has now formally endorsed trauma-informed care, and obstetric guidelines are beginning to include it because trauma histories directly shape outcomes in pregnancy and birth.

But evidence alone doesn't change systems. Culture does. And culture is where patients have power. Every time someone says, "Please explain before you touch me," or "I need you to pause if I raise my hand," or "What are you doing to make this exam trauma-informed?" That's culture mandating change in real time.

Trauma-informed care is not yet the default. But it can be. Until institutions build it in from the top down, the push has to come from us. Patients first, refusing to let trauma be an invisible cost of care.

## Living as a Survivor in Today's Headlines

Right now, it can feel like the world won't let survivors breathe. Whether it's coverage of the Epstein files or the latest high-profile abuse case, you don't have to go looking for it; it finds you. And for so many survivors I talk to, it's not just "news." It's a steady drumbeat of reminders: of what happened to them, of what could have happened, and of how often our society has chosen to protect predators instead of the people they harmed.

You scroll past a headline and your stomach drops. You hear one more expert calmly dissect "what the victims knew" or "what they should have done," and it lands like blame, even if it isn't aimed at you. You watch powerful names emerge from the documents, and the message is depressingly familiar: people with money, status, or proximity to power are buffered in ways survivors never are. It's not partisan. It's cultural. Institutions—from schools and sports programs to churches, hospitals, and courts—have a long track record of circling the wagons around the accused and scrutinizing the people who came forward.

For survivors, that double standard doesn't live in the abstract. It lives in the body. The constant exposure acts like a low-grade reinjury: nervous system on alert, sleep disrupted, old memories jolted awake by each new "exclusive." Even if your own assault had nothing to do with the people in the headlines, the pattern is the same. Someone harmed. Someone protected. Someone disbelieved. And it's hard not to see your own story threaded through that pattern, whether you want to or not.

None of this means we shouldn't report, investigate, or demand accountability. But it does mean we have to name what this moment costs survivors who are just trying to get through a workday, pack lunches, sit through meetings, and schedule their annual exam. You are not "too sensitive" if the coverage leaves you shaky or exhausted. You are not overreacting if you need to mute certain words, log off, or step away from the conversation entirely. Wanting distance from constant reminders of abuse isn't avoidance, it's a form of self-protection.

And here's the piece medicine often misses: when survivors walk into an exam room in the middle of one of these news cycles, they're not starting from zero. They may already be flooded, angry, numb, or on edge before the first question is even asked. If no one in healthcare acknowledges the world we're all living in, we lose a critical chance to make care feel safer instead of like just another place where pain is invisible.

## Medical Training Through a Reproductive Justice Lens

I had the opportunity to interview Loretta Ross, one of the founders of the reproductive justice movement and cofounder of SisterSong, for this book. I asked her what she would change about medical training if she could look at it through a reproductive justice lens. She didn't hesitate. "We brutalize our students and then we expect them to turn around and provide compassionate care. We normalize mistreatment in the training, but then expect them to provide compassionate care."

Her words cut right to the heart of the problem. Healthcare training is ruthless. Long hours. Impossible expectations. Humiliation disguised as "toughening you up." Students are stripped of balance, stripped of compassion, sometimes stripped of their very sense of self, and then expected to walk into exam rooms brimming with empathy. But empathy doesn't grow in environments where humanity is punished. It shrinks. It hardens. And what disappears in training is exactly what patients need most.

## When Providers Carry Their Own Wounds

Loretta's words echoed in me long after our conversation, because I knew what it felt like in my own bones. We don't just brutalize patients in this system, we brutalize providers. We demand resilience while stripping away the very tools that make resilience possible. We demand that students disconnect, suppress, keep moving. We provide no support. And then we're surprised when they lack humanity in the exam room.

When I was in PA school, I had tucked my trauma away. Not neatly—god, no. I didn't realize how much it shaped my anxiety, my depression, my response to stress. I didn't think it mattered. Trauma wasn't covered in my training. I was never screened. Never told that my past might rear its ugly head. And even going into my psychiatry rotation was never warned about what to do if I myself was struggling.

My very first assignment on the rotation? The suicide hotline.

I was immediately triggered. I fought through. As hours crawled on, I was struggling. I couldn't cope. I could barely breathe. That pressure cooker analogy I gave earlier, that was me. I was exploding.

I didn't want to stay there. I couldn't stay there. But I'd been told that missing even one day of a rotation could mean failing it. So I did what so many survivors are forced to do: I white-knuckled my way through it. I panicked. I left early. And in a moment of fear, I falsified my logs, stating that I'd stayed the full day.

I didn't do it to cheat. I did it to survive.

But the truth came out. I was brought before a faculty panel for review. I was forced to stand there, in front of a panel of healthcare professionals, and lay myself bare. My trauma. My mental health. My mistake. I wasn't met with any compassion or care. I was met with punishment.

No one asked what I needed. No one paused to understand what had surfaced, or why. They saw a mistake and decided to make an example of me. I was told I couldn't be trusted. Put on probation. Warned I might not graduate. They told me, point blank, that no employer would want someone "irresponsible" like me. That this would follow me. That my future in medicine was now in question.

A panel made up entirely of clinicians. And not one of them stopped to show even a flicker of concern. Not to ask what I needed. Not to consider the trauma I was carrying. Not to ensure I had support as it flared. Not to consider what it means to stack punishment on top of pain. And certainly, not even to ask the most basic safety question they'd trained me to ask at the suicide hotline: "Are you safe?"

The sheer negligence of that moment still haunts me. These were clinicians. Healers. And yet their response—their anger, their shame, their dismissal—wasn't just a consequence. It was a cruelty. In a moment where my humanity could have been held, I was beaten down.

I lost 15 pounds from the stress. I couldn't eat. I barely slept. My anxiety roared back louder than ever. To this day, I'm still grateful I made it to the other side. Because at that moment, it almost broke me completely.

But here's what I know now:

**My trauma didn't make me a worse clinician. It made me a better one.**

What nearly broke me wasn't the trauma itself. It was the total absence of support when it resurfaced. The expectation that I'd keep pushing forward, like nothing was wrong. As a healthcare clinician in training, the message was clear: don't you dare open that box. Shove it down. Keep going.

I was working in a system that demanded detachment but offered no safety net when my humanity broke through. A training environment that never taught me how to care for patients with trauma, because it never even considered that I might carry some, too.

Clinicians aren't blank slates. We're people with pasts. And people who carry what we've seen. We're the ones who delivered the stillborn. Who watched the fetal heart rate drop and couldn't stop it. Who held the mother's hand when there were no more options. Who carried the look in a partner's eyes when the bleeding wouldn't stop. This work marks us. Sometimes in invisible ways. Sometimes in ways we can't even name until much later.

And yet, we're working in a profession where those traumas are constantly triggered and almost never acknowledged. Medicine teaches us to amputate our emotions. To override our instincts. To perform resilience, even when we're unraveling inside.

But that performance comes at a cost. Not just to us, but to our patients.

In a 2022 dissertation titled "Unacknowledged Trauma: OB-GYNs and the Emotional Impact of Traumatic Birth Events," psychologist Shannon Hensley examined how OB-GYNs process trauma in their own careers—especially around traumatic births, obstetric emergencies, and the kinds of moments that leave you shaken long after you've walked out of the room. She interviewed OB-GYNs across the country. Not one of them said they had received adequate training on how to cope. Not one described formal support. Many admitted they had no language for what they were feeling, only that the impact was real.

Some described sobbing in their cars after shifts. Others talked about numbness, self-doubt, or spiraling anxiety. A few confessed they had considered leaving the field altogether, because the emotional weight was too heavy and there was nowhere to set it down. And still, they went back. They kept showing up for patients. Because that's what the system demands.

But when no one makes space for a provider's trauma, that pain doesn't disappear. It spills. It seeps into the silence. Into the way a provider might freeze when a patient dissociates. Into the moment a clinician goes quiet instead of leaning in. Into the instinct to dismiss, deflect, or detach. Because their own scars haven't been tended to either.

This isn't about blaming providers. It's about recognizing the system-wide silence that's hurting all of us. Because when trauma goes unacknowledged in clinicians, it reverberates back onto patients, especially those who are already most vulnerable.

If a provider seemed cold or distant during your exam . . .

If they shut down when you opened up . . .

If they seemed surprised by your fear, or didn't know what to do with it . . .

It might not have been about you. It might have been about everything they've been taught not to feel.

That doesn't excuse harm. But it helps us understand it. And understanding is the first step toward changing it.

Trauma isn't rare. It's not a niche experience. It's everywhere. Carried in bodies, in exam rooms, in white coats. And the more we allow it to be seen, the less power it has to isolate us. What heals one of us has the potential to heal more of us.

**Your trauma is not a flaw. It's not a weakness. It's a signal, one that deserves to be listened to, not silenced.**

**Our trauma is our superpower.** We can't be told to shove it down. It happened. As horrible as it is, it did. But pushing it down doesn't help. Leaning into it, processing it, unpacking it. *That's* what helps. And it doesn't just help *you*. It helps your provider. It helps future patients. It helps change the room. But the current medical model isn't built for that kind of healing. It isn't set up to hold our stories. It doesn't offer tools for the things that make us human.

Loretta shared with me the aspirational mantra she lives by: "I will always be more than what has happened to me. I will work to become more than my trauma limits me." She reminded me that we can't hand our trauma the remote control to our lives. Because true self-determination means deciding how our story continues. It's not about erasing the past or pretending it never happened. It's about claiming the right to grow beyond it. Healing isn't linear, and it isn't about becoming "fixed." It's about choosing, over and over, to create space for joy, safety, and wholeness in the midst of scars that may never disappear.

We are not machines. We are people. And people carry stories, fear, memory, love, grief, guilt, joy, hope. We walk into exam rooms as whole humans. Even if the system keeps trying to split us apart.

There is nothing shameful about having been hurt. Nothing weak about carrying scars. There is only strength in choosing to see them clearly.

We can't erase the trauma. But we *can* move forward.

# Part Two

# WHEN THE SYSTEM GETS PERSONAL

*From Culture to the Clinic, See How Systemic Failures
Play Out in Everyday Life*

In Part One, we traced the roots of a broken system. From colonization to the classroom and then to the clinic. From blind spots in education to the stranglehold of insurance, from provider burnout to the weight of trauma. We saw how care was built, who it was built for, and the gaps that structure left behind.

Part Two is about the consequences. It's where those systemic flaws show up in the real world. In culture, confusion, misdiagnosis, silence, grief, and growing mistrust. This section names what so many patients have carried alone: the sense that something was wrong, but no one listened.

These stories aren't outliers. They are patterns. And seeing the pattern is powerful.

Part Two connects the dots between the system and the self, naming what so many patients have carried in silence, and creating space for clarity, healing, and a path forward.

# Chapter 8

# When Culture Illuminates the Failures

*How Stories Shatter Silence, Build Community, and Push Medicine to Pay Attention*

Across the board, women want more from reproductive healthcare. We've reached a moment in history where everywhere I look, it feels symbolic of the same truth: we've had enough.

That looks different for every woman. For some, it's refusing to downplay their pain in an exam room. For others, it's naming miscarriage for what it is instead of softening it with euphemisms. For many, it's going public with stories they were once told to hide. Not because they wanted to relive the trauma, but because they knew staying silent would cost someone else even more.

There's a saying I return to often: we stand on the shoulders of those who came before us, and we lay the foundation for those who come after us. Right now, we are sitting in an era where women are realizing that if we don't do something different, it will never get better. Not for us, and not for the ones who come after us. That realization has created a wave of voices refusing to stay silent.

Some are celebrities, speaking openly about their postpartum depression, their infertility, their near-death experiences in childbirth. Some are producers and writers weaving those same truths into the scripts of the shows we binge at night. Some are day-to-day women naming their own reality. Calling into work and saying, without apology or disguise, "I can't come in today because I'm miscarrying." Others are finally saying out loud that their cramps are debilitating, not "just part of being a woman." Others are pushing back against the silence around menopause, refusing to suffer hot flashes, insomnia, and brain fog in shame.

Wherever you turn right now, culture is echoing what women already know in their bones. It's everywhere: on screen, in our feeds, in headlines, in hashtags, and in whispered conversations that grow louder each time someone dares to speak. And those voices don't just create solidarity, they reshape medicine itself. Endometriosis research is finally getting funded after decades of dismissal because patients refused to stay quiet about their pain. Menopause is showing up in documentaries, podcasts, and even corporate wellness programs because women wouldn't keep suffering in silence. Stories force the system to pay attention. And once they're told loudly enough, they can no longer be ignored.

It forges bonds, sometimes trauma bonds, yes, but also bonds of solidarity, of peace, of knowing you were never the only one. And maybe even a hint of hope: that telling the truth might finally move us closer to the care we deserve.

## Trauma and Pain on Screen

One of the most striking places culture has stepped in is through scripted television—dramas that dared to name what medicine minimized. These shows didn't invent pain or trauma; they simply held up a mirror, dramatizing what patients were already living but rarely saw acknowledged out loud.

Take *Grey's Anatomy*. For nearly two decades it has gone beyond love triangles and hospital intrigue, weaving reproductive health into primetime storylines: abortion, infertility, racism in maternal mortality, even menopause. But one episode in particular, "Silent All These Years" (2019), broke open a national conversation. It centered on a woman seeking care after sexual assault, and the writers partnered with trauma experts to make sure every detail rang true. The climactic scene was simple but unforgettable: as the patient was wheeled toward surgery, a long hallway of female staff lined up silently to walk with her. No words, just presence. Just solidarity.

The cultural resonance was immediate. Social media lit up with women saying, *That is me. That is my story*. And the impact wasn't symbolic. RAINN, the Rape, Abuse & Incest National Network, reported a 43% spike in calls to its hotline after the episode aired. A fictional drama had done what medicine so often fails to do: believe women, honor their pain, and create a space where trauma was not minimized, but recognized and carried with compassion.

Enter *The Pitt*, a newer medical drama that pushes those conversations even further. Set in a Pittsburgh ER, the series doesn't tuck health equity into the margins, it places it at the center. Storylines follow a pregnant Black surrogate facing life-threatening complications, a senior Black resident grieving an in vitro fertilization (IVF) miscarriage she may not be able to afford to try again, a teenager nearly denied abortion care because of parental consent laws, and a woman with sickle cell disease dismissed as "drug-seeking" until a culturally competent doctor intervenes. Week after week, patients aren't case studies or teaching moments, they're whole people, carrying histories of bias, barriers, and resilience. By weaving these truths directly into primetime, *The Pitt* builds on what trailblazers like *Grey's Anatomy* have shown us: that medicine on screen can illuminate inequities medicine itself too often erases.

Then there's *The Handmaid's Tale*. What should have been pure dystopia instead became cultural shorthand for reproductive oppression. The red robes and white bonnets spilled from screens into protests across the country. The images of forced exams, coerced births, and women stripped of autonomy felt haunting precisely because they weren't unthinkable, they were eerily close to reality. Patients watching didn't just see Gilead; they saw echoes of their own exam rooms, their own pain waved away as "normal," their own choices narrowed by law or provider bias.

Both shows landed because they named what medicine avoids. They dramatized trauma and pain not as rare "issues," but as daily realities. In doing so, they reminded millions of viewers of something patients have known all along: what hurts the most isn't only the violence itself, but the silence that follows.

## Breaking the Silence About Loss

And it's not just fictional TV. Reproductive healthcare has merged into daily culture and experience as celebrities have publicly and openly shared their experiences. In 2020, Chrissy Teigen shared her family's pregnancy loss on Instagram, posting photos and raw reflections and appropriately using the term *abortion* for spontaneous loss. The reaction was immediate and polarizing. Some questioned her choice to share something so personal, while millions of others thanked her for putting words and images to a grief they had carried in silence. Chrissy and her husband, John Legend, modeled what medicine so often fails to: that naming the truth, even when it's complicated, can help others feel less alone.

That same willingness to bring hidden struggles into the light has shaped other cultural moments, too. Kellie Gerardi, a scientist astronaut and social media creator, has captivated the internet by speaking openly about her infertility struggles, IVF journey, and pregnancy loss. Her candor earned her a Webby award in 2025, proving just how much hunger there is for honesty about reproductive health, and how powerful it can be when someone with a platform gives voice to experiences that medicine often minimizes and society tries to bury. By naming her story, she created space for others to name theirs. What once felt isolating became a point of connection, proof that honesty builds community, and community is what makes support, and change, possible.

## Maternal Health in the Spotlight

Culture has also shined a light on maternal health in ways medicine has failed to. Serena Williams nearly died after giving birth when her concerns about shortness of breath and risk for blood clots were dismissed. Only her persistence, demanding a CT scan and heparin, saved her life. Her story underscored what Black women have been saying for years: their pain is too often ignored, and the consequences can be deadly.

Beyoncé, another of the most visible women in the world, spoke openly about her emergency C-section and her child's stay in the neonatal intensive care unit. Her account made clear that even with immense privilege and resources, she was not insulated from risk. Olympic champion Allyson Felix added her voice when she revealed she lost her sponsorships when she chose to have a child and that she had nearly died from preeclampsia. Her story exposed not only the medical dangers of pregnancy, but the economic penalties of motherhood.

Maternal mental health has entered the spotlight as well. For years, postpartum depression and anxiety were spoken about only in whispers. That began to change when Brooke Shields published her memoir about postpartum depression. More recently, influencers and athletes have spoken candidly about panic attacks, intrusive thoughts, and the crushing weight of loneliness in new motherhood. Their stories reframed postpartum depression and anxiety not as weakness or personal failure, but as the most common complication of childbirth. And one that can be life-threatening when ignored.

These stories did what data could not. The Centers for Disease Control had published maternal mortality statistics for years. Researchers had long documented the prevalence of perinatal mood and anxiety, disorders. But it wasn't until women with platforms spoke out, and spoke plainly, that the public began to listen. By naming their experiences, these celebrities have turned statistics into something far more powerful: a demand for recognition, accountability, and change.

## Identities Made Visible

Culture has also forced visibility for communities medicine continues to overlook. What isn't seen in the exam room shows up elsewhere: on social media, in storylines, and through activism that refuses invisibility.

When Eliot Page, a transgender actor, spoke openly about transition and healthcare, conversations about gender-affirming care—and the routine gynecological needs that don't disappear for trans and nonbinary people—were pushed into mainstream coverage. Hashtags like #TransHealthFail circulated widely, documenting everyday misgendering, denials of care, and retraumatizing exams. What research had long confirmed, that trans patients delay or avoid care because the system isn't built for them, suddenly became visible to millions outside of medical journals.

When fat activists like Tess Holliday and Lizzo called out fatphobia, the conversation about weight bias in medicine shifted out of clinical journals and into cultural consciousness. TikToks about patients being told to "just lose weight" instead of being properly diagnosed went viral, exposing the lazy shortcuts medicine too often takes. The result was cultural accountability: what providers had dismissed as "just advice" was revealed, again and again, as harmful stigma.

When older women refused invisibility onscreen, think Jane Fonda and Lily Tomlin in *Grace and Frankie* sparking conversations about vibrators and sex after 70, it validated what so many had lived but rarely voiced: that aging doesn't erase sexuality, desire, or the right to care. Their presence on screen was more than comic relief; it was a declaration that intimacy and health belong to women at every age.

When disability activists like Alice Wong and the Disability Visibility Project called out inaccessible clinics and broken equipment, they reframed disability from deficiency into identity. Their message was simple but radical: the barriers patients face are not inevitabilities. They are political choices, designed into the healthcare system, and therefore capable of being redesigned.

Together, these stories continue to expose a pattern.

## Cultural Amplifiers of What Medicine Ignores

Sometimes it isn't just individual stories or scripted dramas that break through, it's the megaphone of cultural icons. When someone with a platform as large as Oprah names what medicine has minimized, the effect is seismic.

In 2023, Oprah hosted a televised conversation about menopause that became a cultural turning point. What medical schools had long treated as a footnote, Oprah made headline news. Millions of women tuned in, eager to finally hear their experiences named, validated, and explained. For many, it was the first time menopause had ever been treated as something worthy of primetime.

The conversation was simple but revolutionary: hot flashes, brain fog, sleeplessness, hormone therapy, sex after menopause. Topics that generations of women had been told to "tough out" or accept in silence were suddenly being discussed with the kind of seriousness usually reserved for breaking news. Viewers flooded social media with relief—not because Oprah had discovered something new, but because she had said out loud what so many had been waiting to hear.

That's the power of cultural amplification. When medicine ignores a topic, and culture elevates it instead, the silence becomes impossible to defend. Menopause didn't change overnight. But its place in the cultural conversation did. And that shift matters. It sent a clear message: what medicine relegates to the margins, women know deserves the spotlight.

## Bravery Begets Change

When producers put these stories on screen or celebrities share them with millions, it can feel like culture is changing from the top down. But the truth is, they're responding to something deeper. To what women are already saying quietly in their own lives. They don't invent the narratives; they amplify what has been bubbling under the surface all along.

Because real change doesn't begin on a stage or in a headline. It begins in the quietest places: in kitchens, in break rooms, in text threads with friends, in the moments when we finally admit to ourselves what we've been carrying. Every time an everyday woman hears a story that sounds like hers, she gains a little more permission to name her own truth. That is where change takes root: not just in the spotlight, but in ordinary lives, multiplied until the silence starts to crack.

Storytelling can be medicine. We find healing in hearing our own experiences reflected back to us. We find community in realizing we weren't the only ones. That sense of recognition, of solidarity, can be the first step toward collective change.

And yet, it's important to say this clearly: you don't owe anyone your story. Silence can also be a form of survival, and no one should be forced to speak before they're ready. But if you do choose to share, whether it's with one trusted friend, an online community, or the world at large, know that you're not just freeing yourself, you may be freeing the person listening, too. Multiply that by hundreds, thousands, millions of conversations happening in homes and communities, and suddenly you have momentum. A groundswell. And that momentum doesn't live only online or in headlines. It lives in our daily lives, in the moments when one woman dares to speak and another leans in to listen.

One woman shares her truth at a book club, a church gathering, a workplace lunch, or over coffee with a friend, and suddenly the silence cracks. Her honesty gives permission for others to speak, and soon the conversation is larger than any one person. Just like culture responds to what women demand, communities transform too: each story echoes outward, making it harder for inequities to stay hidden and easier for solidarity to take root. And in exam rooms, too, that ripple matters. When patients come in knowing they are not alone, they bring their truth with less hesitation. And providers are forced to confront realities that can no longer be ignored.

That is how bravery begets change. One voice makes another possible. One story cracks open a door, and another story pushes it wider. And before long, what was once unspoken becomes undeniable. Not because someone at the top decided it mattered, but because women everywhere, at every level, refused to stay silent. And if you carry one thing with you into your next doctor's visit, let it be this: your story and your experience belongs in the room. It is yours to tell, and when you share it, you don't just claim your care, you make more space for the next person to claim theirs, too.

# Chapter 9

# Too Little Time

*Why Short Visits Leave Patients Feeling Unseen and How to Reclaim Your Voice When the Clock Is Against You*

You don't need a primetime drama to know what dismissal feels like. You've felt it. We all have. The rushed visits, the in-and-out pace, the sense that your story was too long for their schedule. Culture may show us the pattern, but the pattern plays out in real life. In the narrow windows we're given to explain our bodies.

In today's system, the time carved out for you is rarely enough. That brief slot is expected to hold everything: bringing up what's happening in your body, asking your questions, absorbing answers, getting examined, and making decisions. All of it crammed into one small appointment, as if care could ever be condensed that way.

So if you've ever walked out of an appointment feeling like you didn't get what you needed—or worse, feeling like you were the problem—you're not imagining it. And you're not alone.

But here's the hard truth: in this system, being a successful patient often means learning how to play a game that shouldn't exist in the first place. You shouldn't have to strategize to receive basic care. But since the system demands it, this chapter is here to help you win.

## When the Visit Ends Too Soon

Short appointments don't just feel unsatisfying, they're dangerous. When the time runs out too quickly, it creates space for miscommunication, for questions left hanging, for symptoms brushed aside. It leaves room for misdiagnosis and missed care. And it leaves patients carrying the medical, emotional, and logistical weight of what didn't get addressed—walking back out the door alone.

Over time, those rushed encounters convince people that the problem is them. That they should've spoken faster, prepared better, or asked differently. That if only they had been clearer, maybe they would've been heard. But let's be clear: this is not about individual failure. It's about systemic design.

When visits are squeezed into narrow blocks of time, providers are forced to prioritize what can be documented and billed, not necessarily what matters most. And in that system, your fear, your grief, your uncertainty, your humanity, is often treated as a time-management problem instead of a legitimate part of your care.

## What Gets Missed in the Rush

The research is clear: shorter visits lead to worse outcomes. And the damage isn't abstract—it's specific, personal, and deeply felt. And let's not forget who's most affected. If you're young, queer, uninsured, disabled, a person of color, or navigating language or cultural barriers, you're even more likely to be rushed, dismissed, or ignored.

This isn't just a coincidence. It's a predictable outcome of a broken system. And we've seen time and time again how it influences medical outcomes.

### Missed Diagnoses

An estimated 5% of US adults experience diagnostic errors in outpatient settings each year. That's 1 in 20 people leaving with something missed, misidentified, or delayed. And most of those aren't zebras. In medical training, we're taught, "When you hear hoofbeats, think horses, not zebras." It's a reminder to consider the most likely, common explanation before jumping to rare diseases. But in reality, what gets missed often are the horses. Things like endometriosis, thyroid conditions, or mental health disorders that don't get enough airtime in a rushed visit. A short appointment. A partial history. No one had time to pause and ask, "What could this really be?"

### Mental Health Gets Skipped

Emotional health rarely fits neatly into a checkbox, and when the clock is ticking, it's usually the first thing to go. But that doesn't mean it's not there. Depression, anxiety, postpartum mood disorders, trauma responses, they often show up in the silence, the body language, the long sighs, and the quiet "I don't know why I'm crying." But if no one asks, and there's no time to say, those concerns stay hidden. And people walk out feeling like they have to carry it alone.

### Superficial Counseling

Whether it's contraception, menopause, hormone-replacement therapy, or antidepressants, treatment decisions require context. They need space for questions, concerns, and follow-up. But when time is short, counseling becomes a checklist: "This is what we usually recommend. Here's your prescription. Let me know if you have issues." Side effects get glossed over. Preferences go unexplored. And when things don't go well? Patients are left wondering if they did something wrong, should have chosen something else, instead of being supported in finding a better fit.

*Unmanaged Chronic Conditions*

From polycystic ovary syndrome to endometriosis to pelvic pain to perimenopause. These are not one-and-done diagnoses. They require sustained attention, nuance, and a care plan that unfolds over time. But short visits break that continuity. Symptoms get dismissed or deprioritized. Labs don't get followed up. And patients are left bouncing between appointments, trying to make sense of it all on their own.

## The Emotional Cost of Being Rushed

I remember a patient at her six-week postpartum visit. On paper, she looked great. Healing well. Blood pressure stable. Bleeding resolved. For billing purposes, the visit was complete.

But before I walked out the door, I asked how she was doing. *Really* doing, and she broke down.

She hadn't slept more than two hours at a time. She was crying daily. She was having intrusive thoughts about something happening to her baby. And she was convinced it meant she was a bad mom.

In a rushed visit, that truth never would've surfaced. She would've sensed there wasn't time, said "I'm fine" and left.

This isn't just about physical health. It's about emotional safety. It's about creating enough space for someone to say, "I'm not okay," and have that admission met with care.

It's about the things patients keep to themselves. Unless someone slows down long enough to ask.

And it's not just postpartum:

- It's the person navigating fertility who smiles through heartbreak because the provider seems rushed.
- It's the patient seeking abortion care who doesn't mention partner pressure because no one asked.
- It's the sexually active teen who gets handed birth control without a single question about trauma.

- It's the trans patient who skips over their symptoms because they can tell the visit isn't a safe place to go deeper.

Across the reproductive landscape, the message is the same:

- If there's no time to ask, the patient stays silent.
- And if it doesn't get asked about, it doesn't get cared for.

That's the real cost of a rushed visit.
Not just what gets missed—but what never even gets offered.

## Where the Time Crunch Hits Hardest: Contraception and Menopause

Two of the clearest examples of how badly the short-visit model fails women's health? Contraception and menopause. On paper, they couldn't seem more different: one is about preventing pregnancy, the other about closing that chapter for good. One often centers young adults just starting out, the other centers people in midlife and beyond. But both expose the same cracks in the system: milestones that deserve time, context, and care get reduced to rushed, surface-level conversations.

And the stakes couldn't be higher. Choosing contraception isn't just about pregnancy prevention. It's about your hormones, your cycles, your sex life, your autonomy. Menopause isn't just about hot flashes. It's about your sleep, your mood, your bones, your heart, and your sense of self. These are not side topics. They are central to health, identity, and quality of life.

Yet these conversations are often treated as optional extras, the first to be brushed aside when the clock is ticking. Symptoms get normalized or dismissed, questions get rushed, and patients are left without clarity or support. Contraception and menopause are just two examples, but they reveal the larger truth: when the system minimizes the very moments that define women's health across the lifespan, it tells us everything about what, and who, it values.

### *Contraception Choice*

Let's start with birth control. In a better world, this conversation would be deliberate and thorough. It would include questions like:

- What are your goals?
- What matters to you about your cycle, your mood, your sex life?
- What have you tried before, and how did it go?
- Are there any concerns about hormones, trauma history, or control?

But more often, here's how it plays out:

"Do you want to stay on the pill?"
"I guess, but I keep forgetting."
"We could do an intrauterine device (IUD)."
"Does it hurt?"
"Just a little cramping. It's very effective."

And that's it. That's the whole exchange. No mention of side effects. No questions about sexual pain or prior experiences with providers. No sense of options, agency, or shared decision-making. Just a recommendation. And out the door.

Don't get me wrong: I love an IUD. Very, very much. But I love it even more when it's chosen after a real conversation. When a patient has the time and space to ask questions, weigh options, and decide it's the right fit; that's when trust begins. That's also when preparation gets better: pain management can be planned, expectations can be clear, and anxiety can be quieted before it spirals. Given enough time, good clinicians do exactly that: they offer options, create space, and support the whole person, not just the uterus in front of them.

The deeper issue is that most contraception counseling skips the part that should be obvious: sex itself. We don't talk about pleasure. We don't talk about comfort. Side effects like dryness, lowered libido, or pain get brushed aside with a "suck-it-up" attitude, as though sexual well-being doesn't matter. It mirrors the broader cultural message women get everywhere else: endure, manage, don't expect too much.

But contraception isn't just about preventing pregnancy. It's about autonomy. Over your health, your choices, your relationships, and your body. And autonomy includes pleasure. Real informed choice means weighing safety *and* quality of life, not treating them as separate. Because your sex life, your comfort, and your well-being are not extras. They are part of the point.

## *Menopause*

Hot flashes. Night sweats. Brain fog. Mood swings. Vaginal dryness. Painful sex. Insomnia. Fatigue.

These aren't small complaints. They're full-body, full-life disruptions. They affect work, relationships, intimacy, sleep, and mental health. And yet, they're often met with little more than a shrug and a "Welcome to getting older."

For many patients, the message is loud and clear: your suffering is normal. It's to be expected. Get used to it. That dismissal leaves people confused, unsupported, and sometimes even embarrassed for bringing it up in the first place. Too many end up questioning themselves, wondering if maybe they really are "crazy," "dramatic," or "ungrateful" for expecting more.

The truth is, menopause is not just a stage of life to be endured. It's a physiological transition that affects nearly every system in the body. Estrogen decline changes bone density, heart health, metabolism, and cognition, not just reproduction. Hormone therapy, lifestyle strategies, and nonhormonal medications exist, but many patients are never told about them. Instead, they're left to suffer in silence, or to Google their way through an overwhelming maze of misinformation and stigma.

Here's the cause and effect: when menopause care is minimized, the result isn't just discomfort. It's missed diagnoses of osteoporosis, untreated depression, worsening cardiovascular risk, preventable fractures, and years of avoidable suffering. Ignoring symptoms today means storing up harm for tomorrow.

And menopause dismissal doesn't exist in isolation, it's part of the broader cultural pattern of brushing off women's pain. Cramps? "Just part of being a woman." Endometriosis? "Probably stress." Painful sex? "Relax more." That lifelong drumbeat of minimization teaches women to doubt their own experience and lowers the bar for what we think we deserve in care. Menopause becomes just another chapter in that same story: one where women's suffering is normalized instead of addressed.

But it doesn't have to be this way. In a better system, menopause would be met with the same attention as any other major health transition. Providers would take symptoms seriously, ask how they're affecting daily life, and walk patients through real options—whether that's hormone therapy, nonhormonal medications, or supportive strategies for sleep, mood, and sexual health. That kind of care doesn't just ease symptoms; it restores dignity. It tells patients their experience matters, that their well-being in midlife and beyond is worth protecting, and that aging should never mean disappearing.

## Building a Care Strategy

You shouldn't need a strategy to get good care, but since you do, let's make sure you're equipped.

This isn't about being a "perfect patient." This is about being a prepared one. It's not fair that this is your responsibility, but learning how to work the system can help you get what you came for.

After navigating my own clinical schedule for over a decade, I can tell you: how a visit is booked *matters*. The visit type matters. The time block matters. Whether the scheduler clicked the right code in the system matters.

Behind the scenes, it changes a lot.

If your visit is scheduled as a procedure, the room gets prepped before you even walk in. The tray is set. The numbing agents are already drawn into syringes. The exact sutures I may need are lined up. The right speculum and vials are pulled out for swabs. Everyone on the team knows what's coming, and they're ready for it.

But if your visit was booked as a quick check-up, none of that happens. Even if *you* show up needing those things, the system wasn't cued to prepare for them. And now we're racing the clock, scrambling to catch up. Scrambling to grab the things we could have easily prepped ahead of time.

Here's how you can advocate for yourself—before you even walk through the clinic doors.

### *Speak Up When Scheduling*

If you have more than one concern—or anything sensitive, emotional, or complex—say that when you make the appointment. Ask if the office offers "extended" or "complex" visits. You might have to wait longer to get the appointment, but it gives you a better shot at securing the time you need.

You can also ask these questions:

- Are there different types of visits?
- Are there providers who offer longer time blocks?
- Is there someone in the practice with specific experience in what I'm dealing with?

Matching with the right provider *and* the right type of appointment from the beginning can set you up for a completely different experience.

### *Know What You Want—And What to Expect*

This one matters more than most people realize. In most practices, not all visits are created equal:

- **Annual exams** are coded as *preventive visits*. They're designed for screenings and quick updates: Pap smears, breast exams, sexually transmitted infection screening, vaccine checks, and

brief birth control refills. What they *don't* cover are in-depth conversations or symptom workups. If you show up with a list of concerns, your provider may not be able to address them at all because of billing rules.
- **Problem-focused visits** are meant for symptoms, questions, or issues you want to dig into. Things like heavy bleeding, painful sex, abnormal discharge, menopausal symptoms, or mood changes.
- **Extended/complex visits** (if offered) give you more time. Ideal if you've got multiple concerns or need to cover something in depth, like fertility planning or a combination of new symptoms.

What does this mean for you? If you've got multiple concerns, it's not an annual preventive visit. If you're struggling with menopause, a deep dive isn't going to happen alongside your Pap smear. That doesn't mean you don't deserve the time. It just means you may need to book more than one type of visit to get what you need.

Be clear with the scheduler about what you're hoping to cover. The more specific you are, the better chance you'll walk into the right room with the right provider, ready to have the right conversation.

## Scheduling Scripts

**If you just need your annual checkup (preventive):**

> "I'd like to schedule my annual preventive exam. This visit is just for my routine screening."

**If you only have concerns/symptoms (problem-focused):**

> "I'd like to schedule a problem-focused visit. I'm having symptoms I'd like to discuss, and I'm not scheduling my annual exam right now."

**If you want both your annual and a separate problem visit:**

"I need to schedule my annual preventive exam, and I also have concerns I'd like to address in a separate appointment. Can you help me book both?"

**If you think you'll need extra time (extended/complex):**

"I have several issues I want to cover, so I want to make sure I have enough time. Does your office offer extended or complex visits?"

**If you're not sure what type of visit you need:**

"I want to make sure I'm scheduled for the right kind of visit. Can you explain what types of appointment you schedule so I can pick the right one?"

## Advocating for Yourself

Your time matters.

Your concerns matter.

And even in a system that wasn't built for you—you *still* deserve to get the care you need.

Until the system catches up, this is how you advocate for yourself. Not because it's fair or right, but because it works.

Here are some strategies to help you get the most from your healthcare.

### *Ask About Telehealth*

Some concerns—like medication refills, follow-up questions, contraception counseling, or menopause support—might be handled just as well (or better) via telehealth. Ask if that's an option. It might make it easier on you.

### *Don't Save the Big Stuff for the End*

The moment your provider walks in, the clock is ticking. Lead with what matters most. Say, "This is my top concern today" or "This might take some time to talk through."

Don't drop an important detail as their hand is on the doorknob walking out.

### *Be Early*

If they ask you to arrive 10–15 minutes early, do it. If you're eight minutes late and they're running on time, you've already wasted a bulk of the time that was reserved for you.

### *Bring Notes*

Write down your questions ahead of time. Use your Notes app or a simple notepad. If your brain blanks under pressure (which is completely normal), your prep will help you stay focused.

### *Bring a Support Person If That Feels Right*

You're allowed to bring someone with you. A partner, a friend, a parent—anyone who helps you feel grounded or supported. They can help ask questions, help you remember what was said, or just be there in solidarity. And if you'd rather go alone? That's valid, too.

### *Know How to Follow Up*

Before you leave, ask how to reach out if more questions come up. Should you use the portal? Call the nurse line? Can you message the provider? Knowing the best way to follow up saves time and helps prevent the frustration of being passed from person to person when you just need an answer.

## Remember: You Deserve More Time

Your concerns are not too much. Your questions are not distractions. Your story is not a burden.

You deserve care that takes the time your body and your life require. You deserve space to feel confused, to grieve, to ask, to process. You deserve providers who treat you as a full person—not a checklist to be completed.

It shouldn't be your job to make a broken system work.

But while we fight for better? You deserve tools. You deserve power. You deserve options.

And if you've ever walked out of an appointment still confused and opened your phone before you even made it to the parking lot?

If you've ever turned to the internet because you *still* didn't know what was going on?

You're not alone.

# Chapter 10

# The Algorithm Will See You Now

*How Social Media Is Shaping the Way We Seek, Share, and Trust Health Information*

A friend of mine went in for a routine ultrasound during her pregnancy—only to be told there was no heartbeat. She got dressed and left the room. She sat in the waiting room alone. For over an hour. No one came in to explain. No one came to offer comfort. No one told her what would happen next.

Eventually, she spoke with a physician, who confirmed the loss, and gave her a vague, clipped rundown. Someone would call her later to go over next steps. But no one called. Not that day. Not the next. Over 48 hours passed before she was referred to a different practice for a dilation and curettage. She wasn't told when the procedure might happen. No one clarified if or when to stop eating. No one explained what to do if she started bleeding at home.

So she went home. Grieving. In shock. Confused. And completely in the dark. And like so many others, she turned to the internet. For clarity, for community, for answers.

Or it's the little things. It's learning more about the birth control options your provider rushed through without context. It's figuring out what your discharge means, or whether your cramps are normal, or whether that medication they mentioned is actually safe to take while breastfeeding. It's discovering that dietary changes might help your polycystic ovary syndrome (PCOS) symptoms. It's something no one in your appointment even brought up.

It's the stuff that should have been part of the conversation in the first place. But wasn't.

## We Were Never Given a Manual

There's this unspoken assumption that we're just supposed to know what to do. That women, especially, come with a user manual for miscarriage, intrauterine device (IUD) complications, side effects, abnormal bleeding, or what to say when something doesn't feel right.

But we don't.

Because no one teaches us.

And it's not traditionally acceptable to talk about.

Comprehensive sex education is barely offered in this country. In 2025, only 36 states and Washington, DC, require it to be taught at all. The United States leads developed nations in teen pregnancy and sexually transmitted infections. States with abstinence-only policies often report even higher teen pregnancy rates.

We're underinformed from the start. And the consequences add up.

Miscarriage is far more common than we're led to believe, affecting about one in five pregnancies. Nearly every pregnant person carries some worry about miscarriage or fetal anomalies. And yet, silence surrounds the reality of it. Most of us aren't told what it might look like, feel like, or mean until we're already in the middle of it—bleeding without warning, waiting for answers, wondering if the cramps are "normal" or if something is dangerously wrong.

We don't know how long the bleeding might last, what medications are available, when to go to the emergency room, or what language to use to get taken seriously. We're handed vague reassurance or outright silence. And so we turn to the internet—trying to solve it ourselves with artificial intelligence (AI), or translating forum posts and Reddit threads into a plan. Grieving, scared, and searching for clarity that should've come from our care team.

And it's not just about fertility or pregnancy. The silence extends well into our 30s, 40s, and 50s. Most people don't know when perimenopause starts, let alone what it looks like. They're blindsided by sleep disruptions, mood swings, painful sex, hot flashes, or weird cycles, without ever being told, "This is hormonal. This is real. This is something you deserve support for."

Instead, it gets brushed off. Or pathologized. Or blamed on stress.

So no, we're not overreacting when we feel lost and alone.

And that's where the internet, and increasingly AI, steps in.

Not because it's ideal.

But because it's there.

## Crowdsourcing Care

The clinic may be the official expert. But the internet is always open. No 10-minute cap. No copay. No checkboxes. People aren't turning to it because it's flawless—they turn to it because care wasn't available when they needed it. And when formal systems leave people rushed, confused, or dismissed, informal ones step in to fill the void. Whether they're helpful or harmful.

And research shows exactly that: patients are most likely to turn to digital platforms when they've been met with stigma, uncertainty, or silence from their providers. That silence isn't always cruel. Sometimes it's just cautious, the quick "let's wait and see" or the jargon-filled brush-off. But the result is the same. People are left piecing together answers from strangers online.

After a miscarriage, for instance, it's often a Facebook group, not a doctor's office, where women first find validation and community.

The scale of this migration is massive. During the pandemic, three-quarters of Americans relied on social media for health information, triple the rate from before, and the habit has stuck. Only 37% of patients now say doctors are their preferred source of health information, while 90% of 18- to 24-year-olds say they would trust medical information shared by peers online. Nearly two-thirds now say they choose providers based on online presence rather than traditional referrals.

Some use these spaces carefully: to fact-check, to crowd-source, to feel less alone. But others get pulled into algorithmic rabbit holes, where influencers with no medical training position themselves as authorities. And when those voices sound more compassionate or more validating than the real-life doctors did, the line between fact and feeling starts to blur. That's where it gets dangerous. Because when expertise feels out of reach, anyone with a confident voice and a camera can claim it. That's how doubt creeps in. Not just about one provider, but about the entire system. And once that trust erodes, it's hard to rebuild.

Nowhere is this clearer than on TikTok. A recent study from La Trobe University analyzed 100 of the most popular TikTok videos on birth control, collectively viewed nearly five billion times. The results were sobering. Only 1 in 10 of those videos were created by a medical professional. The rest came from influencers, self-styled "hormone coaches," or everyday users. More than half rejected hormonal birth control outright. About a third voiced outright distrust in doctors. Fertility awareness and cycle tracking dominated the conversation, while more reliable methods like IUDs or implants barely showed up at all.

The birth-control backlash online didn't just happen. It's been cultivated over years through messaging that deliberately blurs contraception and abortion. Especially emergency contraception and IUDs. That framing shows up in legal language, in public campaigns, in op-eds and "educational" materials, and then seeps into your feed. It's not confusion by accident. Conflation creates fear. Fear pushes people away from the very methods that could help them.

And this matters because the consequences aren't theoretical. When fear wins, fewer people use effective contraception. More unintended pregnancies happen in places with the fewest options. False claims drive vaccine hesitancy. Myths about conditions delay diagnoses and treatment.

And the harm isn't only medical. It's about trust. Once doubt takes root, it changes how we hear everything that comes next. A provider's explanation of the facts can sound like another spin. Even when the clinician is trying to help, it doesn't land the way it should. And once doubt is mixed in, the bond between patient and provider can erode quickly. And it's compounded by the time crunch: with only a few minutes together, too much of the visit gets swallowed up untangling myths from the internet, just trying to get back to baseline, instead of moving forward with a solid plan for care.

That loss of trust is dangerous. It doesn't just affect one appointment or one prescription. If people believe their doctors are withholding the truth, they hesitate before starting birth control. They stop coming back at all. And when large numbers of women lose faith in medicine, it feeds a cycle where misinformation becomes easier to spread and harder to counter, leaving even more people vulnerable.

And here's the bigger picture: contraception has never just been about preventing pregnancy. It has been about freedom. Reliable birth control has been deeply connected to women's ability to pursue education, enter and stay in the workforce, and build careers that once would have been out of reach. It made it possible for women to plan families on their own terms, or to imagine futures beyond motherhood altogether. That freedom reshaped not just individual lives, but families, workplaces, and economies.

So when misinformation chips away at trust in contraception, it's not only threatening someone's immediate health, it's putting decades of progress at risk. The danger isn't just more unintended pregnancies; it's the slow erosion of women's expanded roles in society, a slide back toward a world where they are seen primarily as mothers and caregivers rather than as full participants in every sphere of life.

## The Wild West of Wellness Influencers

But here's the catch: when people go searching for help online, they don't just find facts, they find personalities. Charismatic, confident voices promising answers, healing, and clarity. They find influencers who speak directly to the frustration so many people feel after leaving rushed or dismissive medical visits. "Here's what your doctor won't tell you," they say. "Here's how I healed myself when medicine failed." Some of them mean well. Some are outright grifters. And most are completely unregulated.

This isn't a niche corner of the internet. It's a booming industry. Health and wellness influencers rake in millions selling detox kits, hormone-balancing programs, fertility hacks, and "root cause" testing protocols. Some launch their own supplement lines. Others sell $600 masterclasses and proprietary coaching systems. Many of them brand themselves in soft pastels and spiritual language, creating an aesthetic that feels nurturing and antiestablishment. The surface message is often empowerment, but underneath is a business model that depends on discrediting traditional medicine and offering themselves as the more trustworthy alternative.

And for many people, it works. Not because they're gullible, but because they're tired. Tired of being rushed. Tired of feeling dismissed. Tired of hearing "everything looks normal" when nothing feels normal. These influencers offer something the system often fails to: validation. They speak in plain language, they echo real symptoms, they use emotional tone instead of clinical jargon. They create community, they respond to comments, and they sound like someone who actually *gets it*.

But being compelling is not the same as being qualified. And that's where the danger creeps in. When the person giving health advice has no formal training, no license, and no accountability—but does have a massive platform and a confident tone—it becomes nearly impossible for everyday viewers to tell the difference between science and storytelling, support and sales.

At best, some of these influencers are simply offering benign advice or lifestyle tips. At worst, they are actively spreading misinformation and dissuading people from evidence-based care. Some discourage necessary medications. Others claim to "cure" chronic conditions through restrictive diets, expensive tests, or unproven supplements. Many blend anti-science rhetoric with fear-based messaging, subtly warning followers not to trust their doctors, their pharmacists, or the healthcare system at all.

The consequences are far from theoretical. WHO Europe reports that as much as 51% of social media posts about vaccines, and up to 60% related to pandemics, spread misinformation. Meanwhile, influencers with no medical training regularly push inaccurate claims, often tied to products and profit, not information. This isn't just an issue of bad advice. It's an erosion of trust in real healthcare and what steps in to fill the vacuum when that trust disappears.

Because when patients leave the exam room confused, unheard, or scared, someone will always be waiting online with a more comforting script. And when the system fails to show up with honesty, time, and care—someone else will be there to capitalize on the fallout.

## The Rise of MAHA

One of the clearest examples of how online health conversations grow beyond the screen is MAHA—Make America Healthy Again. Long before it became a political slogan, it was a current on social media: posts about food dyes, seed oils, vaccines, and "overmedicalization" gaining traction through hashtags and wellness influencers.

That online energy didn't stay contained. It translated into a movement with commissions, policy proposals, and a national platform. For many, MAHA resonates because it speaks to real frustrations: chronic illness that feels unexplained, food that feels unsafe, and a healthcare system that too often feels dismissive or out of reach. I can understand why some of its messages land: when you see that certain dyes or additives are banned in Europe but remain common here, the instinct to want cleaner, safer food feels valid.

But side by side with those concerns are narratives built on disinformation. A telling example is the wave of claims about Tylenol use in pregnancy. In MAHA spaces, decades of safe use and clinical research are brushed aside in favor of viral posts suggesting acetaminophen causes autism, attention-deficit hyperactivity disorder, or other neurodevelopmental disorders. Alarming charts and cherry-picked studies get stripped of context, fueling anxiety among pregnant people already navigating a system that often feels uncertain or unsupportive. What begins as a single post questioning "why are doctors still recommending this?" can quickly snowball into a larger narrative that the medical establishment is hiding risks.

The reality is that leading medical groups, including American College of Obstetricians and Gynecologists (ACOG) and the Food and Drug Administration (FDA), still consider Tylenol one of the safest pain relievers in pregnancy when used as directed. But in today's online environment, the nuance of "safe when used appropriately" rarely goes viral. Instead, posts that spark fear, outrage, or certainty tend to rise to the top.

Whether or not you agree with its message, the rise of MAHA shows what happens when conversations that start in Facebook groups and TikTok feeds gain momentum. Social media doesn't just shape individual health choices. It can set the stage for national debates—and even policy.

## The Algorithm Rewards Drama, Not Diplomas

Misinformation spreads because the system behind our feeds rewards the most engaging, not necessarily the most accurate. The algorithm doesn't care about credentials. It's not built to elevate accuracy. It's built to reward engagement. It pushes what performs, not necessarily what's true. The more dramatic, controversial, or emotionally charged the content, the more likely it is to be seen. Outrage spreads faster than nuance. Certainty is more clickable than context. And misinformation wrapped in confidence will outperform nuanced truth.

Social media strategist and influencer Haley Lickstein points out that this isn't accidental, it's algorithmic:

> *"The reality is that women's health has been underresearched and under-discussed for decades, so the stories of being dismissed by a doctor or living with undiagnosed conditions feel painfully familiar. When those stories are shared online, they spread fast. Not because they're accurate, but because they're raw and emotional. Algorithms reward that kind of content. Personal testimony about a dislodged IUD or birth control "ruining your hormones" goes viral because it feels relatable, not because it's true. And once you start engaging with that kind of content, the platforms feed you more of it, trapping you in an echo chamber where those anecdotes start to feel like fact."*

That's why the content that performs best often rises to the top. Even when it's dangerously wrong. There's no fact-checker at the gate, no filter for accuracy before something goes viral. It's not a meritocracy of knowledge, it's a race for attention. And when the algorithm decides what's seen, credibility doesn't always stand a chance.

You can see it everywhere once you start looking. Take the raw milk trend: once a fringe wellness idea, it's now gone viral on

TikTok, packaged in mason jars and pastel aesthetics as "natural" and "pure." It's the perfect example of how misinformation takes hold—because it looks appealing, feels authentic, and travels faster than any correction ever could. Behind the branding, though, is a very real risk: raw milk is far more likely to carry bacteria like *E. coli*, *Salmonella*, and *Listeria*, the very infections pasteurization was designed to prevent.

While the algorithm boosts sensational or misleading content, evidence-based clinicians and creators who offer inclusive, accurate information are often shadowbanned, flagged, or drowned out—especially those discussing abortion, gender equity, or racism. Creators who are Black, queer, or trans face disproportionately aggressive moderation or removal. Research from the Electronic Frontier Foundation shows that abortion-related posts are often shadow banned or de-ranked without warning, even when they comply with platform rules. Creators usually notice only when their engagement suddenly plummets or their accounts vanish from search results unless the full handle is typed in. In one survey of reproductive health-related nonprofits, educators, and businesses, 63% reported content removals on Meta and 55% on TikTok. The very people trying to provide accurate, potentially lifesaving information are silenced at the same time that platforms allow false content to thrive.

This isn't a neutral accident. It's a dangerous double standard. Patients are hungry for credible information, especially in states where abortion and gender-affirming care are restricted or criminalized. But when platforms suppress that information under the guise of "sensitive content," they cut off a critical lifeline. It's an attack not only on reproductive health but also on free expression and the freedom to learn.

And the consequences aren't abstract. Misinformation about contraception changes behavior. It convinces young people that the pill is poison, that fertility tracking is foolproof, or that doctors can't be trusted. When those messages are repeated billions of times, what's at stake isn't just confusion—it's unplanned pregnancies, deepening mistrust, and widening health gaps for the very groups most in need of accurate information.

As the researchers put it, contraceptive misinformation online is reshaping how patients view their doctors, how they make choices, and whether they feel safe trusting medical advice at all.

I saw that erosion of trust in science in my own exam rooms. Patients who once felt confident in their care suddenly questioned everything from their birth control to their doctors' motives. And sure, I'm not saying hormonal contraception doesn't have side effects, It does. But I'd see people who'd been happy on the pill for years, with no issues, wanting to stop altogether while still sexually active and at risk for pregnancy. And it all feels like a massive step backward. The liberation of birth control, this tool that once gave people control over their bodies, education, and futures, is being reframed online as something dangerous or shameful.

And I'm certain that's the point. The growing skepticism around contraception isn't organic, it's engineered. It mirrors a broader effort to erode trust in science, medicine, and bodily autonomy itself. When misinformation spreads under the glossy language of "wellness" or "natural living," it doesn't just sell products, it reshapes beliefs. It convinces people they're reclaiming control by rejecting modern medicine, when in reality, they're being guided toward choices that make pregnancy more likely and options more limited. In a moment when access to abortion and comprehensive reproductive care is already shrinking, that coincidence feels less like chance and more like strategy.

It's subtle. It doesn't look like control being taken. It looks like freedom being offered. But that's the deception of it. It isn't just misinformation; it's manipulation. A quiet reprogramming of public belief that trades real autonomy for the illusion of it. The loss of trust isn't accidental. It's the mechanism that makes control look like choice.

## When Hashtags Become Your Healthcare Plan

This is what people seek out when they leave a rushed appointment with questions unanswered. It's not that they think the internet is better than their doctor. It's that they don't have the access to their doctor that they do with the internet.

And, yes, they're looking for information. But they're also looking for connection. For someone to say, "I've been through this, too." For a thread that feels like a lifeline when everything else has gone quiet. For a comments section that they can see themselves in.

Most users know what they're reading online might be flawed. 77% say they're skeptical of health trends they see on social media. But they still rely on them. Because they don't have another option. Because something is better than nothing.

When it comes to miscarriage and fertility, social media isn't just noise, it's often a lifeline. Platforms like Instagram have become vital spaces for support, solidarity, and visibility. Women grieving loss post with raw honesty. Strangers reply with empathy, understanding, shared grief. That communal load sharing, the emotional, practical, and even medical talk, isn't incidental; it's therapeutic.

But those posts also underscore what's missing offline: clear counseling, compassionate explanations, reliable education. In a world where the medical system often retreats into silence or jargon, social media becomes the vent, the voice, the virtual hand reaching out to say, "I see you, and you're not alone."

It's not that people don't want to get their information from medical professionals. Most would prefer it. But many have stopped believing they'll get the full story. Get the time they need. Get the real answers, the real solutions.

Declining trust in science, political polarization, and deep-rooted medical racism and sexism have all contributed to this mistrust. Even when patients do come in prepared, with questions pulled from TikTok or Reddit or research of their own, they're often met with defensiveness. Dismissiveness. Condescension. And that only deepens the divide.

And that divide has consequences.

## The Real Cost of Bad Information

The damage ripples outward. Misinformation fractures families, divides communities, and erodes the foundation of shared truth. It spreads faster than corrections, sticks harder than facts, and thrives in digital spaces that reward confidence over accuracy. Health misinformation changes behavior.

It convinces people to skip vaccines, avoid necessary medications, or try dangerous remedies they found online. It fuels disordered eating patterns wrapped in wellness language. It spreads myths about fertility, birth control, and disease prevention. It delays care, not just for minor issues, but for life-threatening ones, because people are left unsure whom to trust or what to believe.

And the harm is real. Not abstract. Not academic. Tangible, measurable harm. Fear. Confusion. Emotional exhaustion. Burnout. For patients trying to piece together a care plan and for providers trying to combat myths that feel louder than science.

Because when people are constantly second-guessing their symptoms, their providers, and themselves, it becomes harder to advocate, harder to heal, harder to access care at all. And when providers are forced to spend precious time unraveling internet-fueled fears instead of treating the person in front of them, everyone loses.

This isn't just a social media problem. It's a systems failure.

## From Google to ChatGPT: The New Frontline of Care

For years, the first stop after a confusing symptom has been Google. Stomach pain, weird discharge, headaches that won't quit. Millions of us type our worries into a search bar and brace ourselves for the results. Sometimes it's helpful. Sometimes it's a rabbit hole of contradictory advice and worst-case scenarios. Either way, it's become part of the ritual of seeking care: look it up online first, then decide if it's "serious enough" to call the doctor.

Now that habit has taken a leap forward. Instead of a list of links, AI tools like ChatGPT talk back. They don't just give you articles, they generate answers, translate medical jargon into plain language, and even mirror the tone of a compassionate provider. For someone who's been dismissed in the exam room, that feels groundbreaking. Suddenly, a tool is listening, responding, and validating the concern.

But here's the catch: AI doesn't "know" in the way a clinician does. It predicts text based on patterns, not diagnoses based on training. Sometimes the answers are accurate and empowering; sometimes they're misleading or flat-out wrong. And because AI delivers everything with confidence, it can be easy to mistake plausibility for truth. For a patient sitting at home after a miscarriage or chest pain, that confidence can comfort or dangerously mislead.

There are privacy risks, too. Every symptom typed into a chatbot becomes data, with little transparency about how it's stored or used.

Still, the trend is undeniable. Millions are already turning to AI for answers. It's not because people believe chatbots are perfect. It's because they're desperate for clarity and the system didn't give it to them. AI isn't replacing doctors. It's replacing silence. Just like social media, it fills the void left when the health system fails to explain, guide, or support.

## So, What Do We Actually Do About It?

This chapter isn't about criticizing people for going online. It's about understanding why we had to, and helping to do it more safely. People aren't searching online because they're reckless or lazy. They're there because they're desperate for answers, for connection, for clarity.

Because when you walk out of a clinic with more questions than you came in with, the internet is the next place to go. That isn't a moral failing, it's a reflection of need.

The truth is, not all providers understand the online world their patients live in. Many haven't been trained to communicate in plain language. They don't always know how to explain complex issues without jargon, or how to validate someone's experience without minimizing it. And the systems they work in often don't give them the time or resources to do better. That disconnect leaves patients on their own, trying to translate medical uncertainty into something they can actually understand.

And here's the part that's worth saying out loud: the confusion about reproductive healthcare online didn't just happen by chance. It's been cultivated over years through language that blurs and distorts—equating contraception with abortion, framing miscarriage management as criminal, or casting fertility treatments as suspect. These narratives have been used in courtrooms, in legislative debates, and in public campaigns. And once those frames take hold, they don't stay confined to politics, they trickle into everyday conversations, into exam rooms, and into the feeds we scroll at night. That's why you'll see claims that IUDs "cause abortion," that the morning-after pill "ends a pregnancy," or that in vitro fertilization is inherently unsafe. Those aren't random myths. They're the fallout of deliberate efforts to sow doubt, and they leave patients questioning care that is safe, evidence-based, and often essential.

But you can learn to spot red flags in health content online. You can learn how to fact-check claims that sound convincing but aren't backed by evidence. You can bring notes to your appointment. Ask follow-up questions. Say when something doesn't make sense. You can claim space in the exam room, even if the system isn't built to offer it freely.

And at the same time, healthcare spaces need to meet you there. Providers and institutions must begin acknowledging the influence of digital platforms. Not just as a source of misinformation, but as a place where trust can be built, too. Dismissing everything online as "bad information" misses the point. If patients are turning to social media, or even AI chatbots like ChatGPT, before or after they turn to their provider, then that's where care conversations are already happening. Ignoring that reality only deepens the divide.

There are better ways to search. Smarter ways to advocate. And small, practical steps you can take, right now, to stay informed, safe, and connected.

## A Better Way to Search

Until the system improves, people will keep searching. And that's okay. This isn't a call to stop searching online, it's a call to do it smarter. Because while it shouldn't fall on patients to fact-check their own care, the reality is that it often does. But with the right tools, you can approach online information with more confidence, clarity, and caution.

No one should have to become their own doctor just to feel heard. But until the system catches up, learning to navigate the noise is a form of protection. A way to take back some control. You don't have to know everything. You just have to know enough to ask better questions, and refuse to settle for silence.

### *Start with Strong Sources*

When you're researching anything health-related, begin with sites that cite peer-reviewed studies, medical institutions, or public health organizations. Names like the Mayo Clinic, Cleveland Clinic, Johns Hopkins, ACOG, the Centers for Disease Control, and the World Health Organization are usually safe places to start. Be cautious with websites that make big claims but don't cite where their information came from. If a site doesn't list sources, references vague studies without links, or sells a product, that's a red flag.

### *Use AI Tools Wisely*

Think of them as prep, not prescription. Use them to brainstorm questions, to make complex information easier to understand, or to give you language to bring into an appointment. Don't use them for emergencies, and never treat them as a final diagnosis. Always cross-check what you get with a trusted provider.

### *Remember: Trending Doesn't Mean True*

The internet prioritizes engagement, not accuracy. Algorithms reward clicks, controversy, and confidence, not credibility. That influencer who seems so sure about hormone-balancing powders or anti-vaccine conspiracies may have no training at all. Always ask yourself, *Is this person providing education or entertainment?*

### *Look for Consensus, Not Just Confirmation*

If something sounds new, surprising, or drastically different from what you've heard elsewhere, dig deeper. One post, one reel, one blog, or one AI-generated answer, is never the full story. Reliable medical guidance usually doesn't swing wildly. It builds slowly, with research and peer review. The best health advice tends to be boring, steady, and consistent across multiple platforms.

### *Save Your Questions and Bring Them with You*

If something you read online raises a question or gives you pause, don't dismiss it. Screenshot the post, write it down, or keep a list in your Notes app. Bring it to your appointment. A good provider won't be offended or annoyed, they'll be glad you care enough to ask. And if they're dismissive or condescending? That's not your fault. You're allowed to find someone who respects your curiosity and takes the time to explain.

### *Trust Your Instincts, but Verify the Details*

You know your body better than anyone else. If something feels off, it probably is. That gut feeling is worth listening to. But make sure the path you take in response is grounded in evidence, not just anecdotes, opinions, or marketing. Especially when it comes to supplements, hormone therapies, or anything that could affect your health long-term—double-check the science before you act.

### *Give Grace to Yourself and to Others*

This system isn't easy to navigate. It withholds information, uses inaccessible language, and too often makes people feel small for not already knowing what they were never taught. If you've ever felt behind or overwhelmed, you're not alone. You're not doing it wrong. In fact, the fact that you're even reading this means you're already doing more than most. You're learning. You're showing up. You're trying to take ownership of your health in a system that hasn't made that easy.

# Chapter 11

# When Your Voice Isn't Enough: Gaslighting, Bias, and Discrimination in Care

*The Systemic Failures That Silence Patients and the Tools You Need to be Heard*

**W**e've already talked about what happens when patients leave appointments with more questions than answers. About the endless Googling, the TikTok deep dives, the late-night Reddit scrolls. Because the system didn't give them what they needed.

But sometimes, you figure it out. You find the right language, the right research, the right diagnosis. You come in prepared. Symptoms tracked, studies saved, story straight.

And still, you're dismissed.

This is what happens when you come in informed, and your provider doesn't listen. When they tell you it's all in your head.

When the tone shifts. When you start to doubt what Start you know to be true.

That's medical gaslighting. And it's a lot more common than most people realize.

Medical gaslighting is when a healthcare provider dismisses, downplays, or questions your symptoms in a way that causes you to second-guess your own experience. It can sound polite. "That's just part of being a woman." Or patronizing. "You've probably been reading too much online." Either way, the impact is the same: it undermines your trust in your body, your voice, and your instincts.

It isn't just a frustrating experience. Medical gaslighting is now recognized as a top patient safety concern in America. A major 2025 patient safety report found that 94% of patients have experienced having their symptoms dismissed by providers. Even more alarming: over half of those patients said their symptoms got worse after being dismissed, and 28% ended up having a health emergency because their concerns weren't taken seriously.

## What Medical Gaslighting Looks Like

Medical gaslighting is what happens when your very real concerns get brushed aside without proper evaluation, whether because of a provider's ignorance, bias, or just plain medical paternalism. It doesn't always come from cruelty or malice. Most clinicians don't set out to harm. But the effect is the same: you walk away doubting yourself. You wonder if the pain is "in your head," if you're being "dramatic," if maybe your body isn't telling you what you thought it was.

When I was in clinical rotations, one of my preceptors gave me advice I've never forgotten: "Sit down and shut up."

He meant it kindly. "If you just let them talk, patients will tell you what's wrong. You just have to listen."

Such a simple idea, and yet so radical in practice. Because the truth is, we don't actually train clinicians to trust patients. We train them to control the visit, check the boxes, and filter the story through a clinical lens. But diagnoses don't always look like they do in textbooks.

## The Science of Being Silenced

The truth is, most doctors don't have the time, training, or even the mindset to slow down and really listen. And we're not just talking about a bad day or one rushed appointment. This is a systemic issue.

Studies show that physicians interrupt patients almost immediately. One study found that doctors cut patients off after a median of just 11 seconds. And some jumped in as quickly as 3 seconds after the patient started talking.

But when patients *aren't* interrupted? They usually finish what they have to say in well under a minute, an average of 46 seconds. That's it. Yet even that window is rarely given.

## The Reality of Dismissed Pain

The word *hysteria* comes from the Greek word for *uterus*. For centuries, "female hysteria" was a catch-all diagnosis for women who dared to show too much emotion: anxiety, anger, even sexual desire. The diagnosis may be gone, but the mindset it left behind still echoes through today's exam rooms. Women's pain is often minimized, dismissed, or reframed as exaggeration, hormones, or imagination.

That dismissal is not abstract. It shows up in measurable ways. In one emergency department study of nearly 1,000 patients with acute abdominal pain, women were less likely than men to receive pain medication (60% versus 67%) and waited longer to get it. 65 minutes compared to 49. Women reporting chest pain waited 29% longer to be evaluated for heart attacks. Even when they reported the same pain levels as men, they were still less likely to receive relief. In one study, only 38% of women received pain medication compared to 47% of men with identical symptoms. When nurses reviewed identical case vignettes, with patients rating their pain as 9 out of 10, they consistently rated the man's pain higher than the woman's. Same pain. Different assumptions.

Across the world, across hundreds of conditions, not just reproductive ones, women are diagnosed years later than men. A Danish study of 6.9 million people found that, on average, women received the same diagnoses about four years later than men did. Cancer was diagnosed 2.5 years later, and metabolic diseases like diabetes were diagnosed 4.5 years later. Follow-up research confirms this disparity holds across more than 100 acute and chronic diseases, spanning over 208 million patients, where women consistently face longer delays to diagnosis than men, even when presenting the same symptoms.

Researchers are still unraveling whether biology, environment, provider bias, or all three are at play. The difference is significant. As lead author Søren Brunak pointed out, men generally go to the doctor later than women, so the gap in onset may be even wider. That means by the time a woman's symptoms are taken seriously, she's already years behind in treatment.

The problem is not limited to sex or gender. Racial bias compounds the dismissal of pain. Black women in the United States are systematically undertreated compared to white patients. In one study of more than one million emergency department visits, Black patients were significantly less likely than white patients to receive opioid pain treatment for the same conditions. And research has shown why: many medical trainees and providers still hold false beliefs about biological differences between Black and white patients, beliefs that lead directly to disparities in pain assessment and treatment. For Black women, those racial biases often layer onto the broader gendered dismissal of pain, creating a double burden.

This is the legacy of hysteria, embedded into modern practice: men in pain are still coded as "stoic," while women are coded as "dramatic" or "emotional." And when race, class, or sexuality are layered on top, the dismissal becomes even more entrenched. These biases are not just attitudes, they translate into delayed diagnoses, undertreatment, and unnecessary suffering. It's baked into the system. And it's still hurting people every day.

## The Hidden Curriculum of Bias

Medical bias isn't always loud or obvious. It doesn't just show up in the way a doctor talks to you. It starts much earlier, in medical training. Doctors don't only learn from textbooks; they pick up habits, shortcuts, and attitudes from the doctors who train them. This "hidden curriculum" gets passed down quietly, without anyone ever saying, "This is bias."

Take one example: the six Fs. It's a mnemonic taught to medical students to remember who is most at risk for gallstones: fat, fertile, forty, female, fair, and family. Easy to memorize, sure, but also loaded with stereotypes. When trainees are taught to link disease risk to body size, gender, or even skin tone, those assumptions can stick. Instead of listening carefully to a patient's individual story, a provider may unconsciously slot them into a stereotype. That can mean missed diagnoses or delayed care.

And it isn't just old sayings. Many of the medical algorithms that doctors rely on—tools that guide decisions about who gets tested, who gets treated, and how urgently—are built on biased data. If the data came from mostly white, male patients, then the "science" will quietly encode those same gaps. The result? A patient who doesn't fit that mold might get overlooked.

Even new technology isn't solving this problem. Half of the artificial intelligence (AI) systems being used in healthcare show bias against women and people of color, often because they're trained on data from mostly white, male patients. So the same patterns get baked into supposedly "objective" computer systems.

On top of that, medical students learn by watching. If they see senior doctors brushing off women's pain, making assumptions about Black patients, or blaming fat patients for their health concerns, that becomes their norm. Bias isn't always taught directly, it's absorbed.

And here's the kicker: a third of medical trainees let race or gender shape their treatment decisions, and half of them didn't even realize they were doing it. That's what makes it so dangerous. Bias doesn't always announce itself as bias; it hides under the cover of "good medicine," disguised as clinical judgment. But when it goes unrecognized, it doesn't just influence one decision, it gets steeped into training, passed down to the next class of providers.

## The Reality of Overlooked and Misunderstood Conditions

Gaslighting doesn't just happen one-on-one in exam rooms. It's embedded in the way our entire medical system is structured, especially when it comes to conditions that don't show up cleanly on labs, imaging, or quick diagnostic checklists.

Take vulvodynia. It often presents as burning, rawness, stinging, or knife-like pain in the vulva. It is sometimes constant, sometimes triggered by something as simple as sitting, wearing tight clothing, or attempting sex. The pain can make intimacy difficult, complicate basic daily activities like exercise or even walking, and chip away at a person's sense of normalcy and self. Despite being recognized by the National Institutes of Health and studied for decades, women reporting chronic vulvar pain are frequently dismissed, told it's "in their head," or misdiagnosed altogether. In one qualitative study, women described repeated invalidation by providers who minimized their pain, questioned their credibility, or lacked even basic knowledge of the condition.

And vulvodynia isn't the exception. This pattern repeats across a wide range of so-called contested illnesses, conditions that are real, researched, and deeply felt by patients, yet still debated or dismissed in clinical, legal, and public discourse.

The harm is not abstract, it's lived every day. People with dyspareunia (painful intercourse), fibromyalgia (widespread pain with fatigue and brain fog), chronic pelvic pain, or dysmenorrhea (severe menstrual cramps) are often told their suffering is "subjective" or "inconclusive"—a medical euphemism for "we don't know what to do with you." In a study of women with fibromyalgia, that kind of invalidation wasn't just frustrating; it was directly linked to poorer quality of life and lower trust in medical care.

Not knowing how to help is one thing. Suggesting nothing is wrong is another. And far too often, patients with these conditions hear exactly that. Many leave appointments feeling stunned, ashamed, or gutted after being dismissed by the very people they trusted for care. Some stop seeking help altogether. Others turn the blame inward, losing trust not just in their providers but in themselves.

One of the most common labels applied in these situations is medically unexplained symptoms (MUS). On paper, it sounds neutral. A placeholder until more evidence is found. In practice, though, it often becomes shorthand for "we don't see it, so it must not be there." The term frequently blurs into another label, *psychosomatic*, which implies symptoms are "all in your head." Neither is inherently meant to dismiss patients, but that's how they land. Because many of these conditions *do* have diagnostic criteria, research, and evidence behind them, yet the MUS or psychosomatic label gets applied anyway, shutting down investigation before the real work begins. For patients, it can feel less like a medical assessment and more like a judgment: "You're imagining this." And that feels a whole lot like gaslighting.

To be clear, mental health, stress, nutrition, and lifestyle absolutely influence our physical well-being. But when those explanations are offered without proper evaluation—when someone's symptoms are chalked up to weight, anxiety, or "just being a woman"—it sends a dangerous message: that the illness is your fault. Or worse, that there's no illness at all.

## The Real-World Impact: When Trust Breaks Down

Gaslighting in healthcare isn't just frustrating, it's dangerous. Patients who feel dismissed are more likely to delay appointments, underreport symptoms, or avoid care altogether. Over time, that self-doubt can snowball: *Maybe I really am overreacting?*

Research consistently shows that when patients feel heard and respected, health outcomes improve. People are more likely to follow treatment plans, seek preventive care, and engage actively in their health. Conversely, surveys show that many leave clinical visits feeling ignored. One national poll found that 52% of US adults report their symptoms are dismissed or disbelieved by providers. Another survey found that over 70% of adults believe the healthcare system is failing them in at least one way.

Feeling unheard doesn't just sting, it shifts the entire trajectory of care. When trust erodes, people delay appointments, ignore symptoms, and wait too long to seek help. What gets lost in that gap isn't just time. It's health. It's safety. It's lives.

## What Actually Doesn't Work

Here's what research tells us doesn't work: mandatory training about bias. Study after study shows that even extensive bias training, averaging more than five hours per provider, doesn't actually change how doctors treat patients in the long run. Awareness might increase, but behavior stays the same.

Other reviews have found similar patterns: implicit bias trainings can make providers more *aware* of stereotypes or even more confident that they've "checked the box," but they rarely shift the structural pressures or daily habits that shape real-world care. At worst, mandatory trainings can backfire, provoking defensiveness, reinforcing stereotypes, or creating a sense of fatigue for equity work.

And I've seen it firsthand. In Michigan, the state now mandates that every clinician complete one hour of implicit bias training for license renewal. On paper, it sounds promising. In practice,

I watched colleagues log into a virtual training, mute it, and let it run in the background just to check the box. The requirement was met, the certificate printed, but nothing in the room, or in the exam room that followed, had actually changed.

The evidence is clear: bias is not something you can lecture away in a classroom or fix with a certificate. It's embedded in policies, workflows, and incentive structures. Things much bigger than any individual training module. Without systemic change, providers return to the same rushed visits, the same billing codes, and the same unconscious shortcuts that lead to unequal treatment.

## Strategies for Navigating Bias, Gaslighting, and Discrimination

No matter what kind of barrier you're facing, whether it's being dismissed in the exam room or excluded by the system before you walk in, a few strategies always help. Prepare before your visit, be clear during it, and document afterward. Bring someone you trust when you can, and remember: it's not a failure if you need to seek a second opinion or switch providers. That's part of advocating for yourself.

From there, the specifics of how you navigate depend on the challenge in front of you.

### When You're Gaslit: Strategies for Being Heard

Being dismissed in the exam room can shake you to your core. It's not just about not getting answers in the moment, it's about the way it makes you question yourself. Was I overreacting? Did I make too much of this? That self-doubt is exactly what gaslighting breeds, and it's why having strategies in your pocket matters. The goal isn't to fight your provider, it's to keep your footing when the ground starts to feel shaky, and to make sure your concerns don't get lost in the shuffle.

### Before Your Appointment: Set the Stage

Walk in ready, not reactive. Write down your symptoms and concerns, a few bullet points on your phone or a notepad is enough. Track patterns that matter: pain that comes and goes, fatigue tied to your cycle, symptoms that disrupt sleep, work, or relationships. Think of it as a road map, not to do your provider's job but to make it easier for them to see the full picture.

And yes, you're allowed to research. You don't need to arrive with a diagnosis, but you can ask questions such as these:

- "I've been reading about [X]. Could this be worth exploring?"
- "What would it look like to rule that out?"
- "Is this something that could be contributing to my symptoms?"

You're not being difficult. You're being engaged.

### During Your Appointment: Keep Your Power

If the pace feels too fast, pause with "I need a moment to process that."

If options feel limited, ask "What are all my choices?" or "What should I expect from this treatment?"

If you're brushed off, redirect with "What else could be going on?" or "Can you explain why this isn't concerning?"

These phrases slow things down, open space, and remind your provider that your understanding matters.

### Bring Backup

Appointments can be overwhelming. Bring a partner, friend, parent. Anyone who can ask questions, take notes, or speak up when you need a breath. If no one can come, request a visit summary or access your records afterward. You're legally entitled to have someone with you if you want, and we'll touch on that in a bit.

*After the Appointment: Stay in Control*

Document everything. Follow up if something wasn't clear. If you left feeling dismissed, again, it may be time for a second opinion. That's not failure. That's strategy.

## When the System Excludes You: Strategies for Navigating Discrimination

Bias isn't always subtle. Sometimes it's built into the very structure of care: the wrong-size blood pressure cuff, the intake form with no box for your identity, the inaccessible exam table, the provider who won't look you in the eye. Other times it's the quieter slights. The assumptions, the stereotypes, the policies that were never designed with you in mind. Facing discrimination in healthcare isn't about one bad interaction, it's about a system that wasn't built for all of us. These strategies won't fix that system on their own, but they can help you protect your health while we keep pushing for change.

*Before the Appointment: Research and Prepare*
- **Find affirming providers:** Look for clinics that advertise LGBTQ+-affirming, fat-positive, trauma-informed, or disability-accessible care. Read reviews. Ask your community.
- **Prepare for barriers:** Call ahead about equipment, parking, or interpreter services.
- **Know your rights:** Learn antidiscrimination protections under the ACA, Section 504, and your state laws.
- **Share your needs:** If you'll need a larger gown, accessible exam table, interpreter, or a trauma-informed approach, tell the office ahead of time.

*During the Appointment: Assert Your Needs*

- **Be specific:** Don't assume providers know what you need. Say clearly if you want to skip the scale, state your pronouns, or need extra processing time.
- **Bring documentation:** Have a list of symptoms, questions, and medications to keep the conversation anchored.
- **Use advocacy support:** A friend, doula, or partner can not only support you emotionally but also serve as a witness if bias arises.

*After the Appointment: Hold Systems Accountable*

- **Document discrimination:** Keep notes of what happened, who was involved, and how it affected your care.
- **Seek alternative care:** You can leave mid-visit. You can change providers. If care was unsafe or discriminatory, you deserve better.
- **File complaints:** Report issues to the clinic, hospital, licensing board, or the Office for Civil Rights. Keep in mind, it's not just about your care. It protects the next person, too.

*Beyond Your Visit: Why the System Needs to Change*

Even the best preparation can't fix a system built for a narrow slice of people. That's why self-advocacy matters, but it's not enough. We need the following:

- **Policy that protects patients:** Enforceable nondiscrimination standards, inclusive intake forms, accessible equipment
- **Training that actually changes practice:** Ongoing education in structural racism, LGBTQ+ health, fatphobia, disability justice, trauma-informed care
- **Data that doesn't disappear us:** Outcomes tracked and published by race, gender identity, income, disability

- **Care that comes from community:** Black-led birth collectives, queer health centers, disability justice networks often provide models rooted in trust and equity

## Holding Your Ground

Self-advocacy isn't about being perfect. It's about asking uncomfortable questions, holding your ground when something feels off, and refusing to shrink just because someone else won't make space. You don't need permission to take up that space. You deserve to be heard.

Gaslighting isn't just frustrating, and discrimination isn't just inconvenient. Both are dangerous. They cost time, trust, and lives. When patients come in prepared, clear about their symptoms, and still aren't believed, the harm compounds. Dismissal becomes delay. Delay becomes misdiagnosis. And misdiagnosis can become something much worse.

But knowledge is power. Recognizing patterns, preparing for appointments, asserting your needs, and building support for your care can give you back some control. It won't fix a broken system, but it can help you move through it with more clarity, more confidence, and more safety.

And with enough of us speaking up, sharing our stories, and refusing to be silent, the pressure on the system will only grow. Until one day, being heard won't be the exception. It will be the baseline. The bare minimum. Exactly what everyone deserves.

## Bringing Backup: How to Ask for the Support You Need

You don't have to navigate this system alone. If you have a partner, friend, parent, or loved one who's willing to show up for you, here's what support can look like and how you can communicate the help you need.

A support person doesn't have to be a medical expert. Their role is simple: to hold space, to back you up, and to make the appointment feel less overwhelming. You can ask them to do the following:

- Take notes so you can stay present.
- Remind you of questions you wanted to ask.
- Speak up if you're being rushed or dismissed.
- Simply sit beside you so you don't feel alone.

If you're not sure how to ask, here are a few ways to phrase it:

- "It would help me if you could take notes during the visit so I don't forget anything."
- "If I freeze up, could you ask this question for me?"
- "Can you just be there and help me process afterward?"

Support can also go beyond the exam room. You might ask someone to call ahead about accessibility, help you research affirming providers, or keep track of what happened if you experience discrimination. Sometimes the biggest gift is having someone else carry part of the weight.

You don't need to feel guilty for asking. Needing support doesn't make you less capable, it makes you human. And the right person will want to help. The hardest part is often just naming what would make you feel seen and safe.

# Part Three

# YOUR BODY, YOUR VOICE

*From What's Broken to What's Possible*

In Part One, we exposed the cracks in the system. How poor training, profit models, and systemic bias shape the care we receive. In Part Two, we traced the lived consequences. How those cracks show up in our bodies, our lives, and our trust.

Now, we shift. Part Three is what you can do about it.

The system may not change overnight, but how the way you navigate it can.

This section is about finding your voice and using it. Not to shout over a system that doesn't hear you but to steady yourself within it. To walk into appointments with language, tools, and self-trust that you may not have had before.

It's not about becoming your own doctor. It's about becoming your own advocate.

And knowing that your needs, your boundaries, your voice, were never "too much."

They were never extra. They were necessary. Now let's channel them.

# Chapter 12

# Learning Your Body and Your Needs

*You Can't Advocate for Yourself if You've Been Taught to Ignore Your Body; Let's Change That*

Most of us never learned how to actually know our own bodies. We were taught how to hide them, shrink them, fix them. How to ignore what they were trying to tell us. And after years, sometimes decades, of that messaging, it's no wonder people walk into medical appointments without the words to describe what they're feeling. Not because they're clueless or careless. But because they were never taught how to listen.

This chapter isn't just about being your own advocate. It's about rebuilding trust with yourself. It's about noticing the signals your body sends, honoring those signals, and saying them out loud. Without shame or apology. The healthcare system isn't built to ask the right questions, so you have to bring your own clarity into the room.

Clarity doesn't come from a checklist. It starts inside you. Self-advocacy isn't a performance. It's a practice rooted in *awareness*.

In *curiosity*. In your own willingness to pause and ask yourself these questions:

- *What am I feeling?*
- *What have I learned to ignore?*
- *What does my body need right now?*

Before you can speak up for yourself, you have to be able to hear yourself.

## When Disconnection Becomes the Default

Let's name it: many of us have been taught to disconnect from our bodies.

We learn early to downplay discomfort, to tolerate pain, to explain away symptoms with phrases like "it's probably nothing." We get called *dramatic, sensitive,* or *too much*. We get praised for being "low maintenance." For not needing anything, for not making a fuss. For ignoring our own needs to make other people comfortable.

Or, we never learned how to connect in the first place. We don't know how to check in with our bodies. How to name hunger or fatigue *before* getting hangry. How to tell the difference between anxious and excited *before* it spiraled into a panic attack. We may not have honed what it looks like to listen inward.

When you live in a body that's been judged, objectified, policed, or pathologized, when your body has been treated like a problem to solve or a thing to fix, disconnection can become second nature. Maybe your body was commented on more than it was cared for. Maybe your feelings were brushed off, or your symptoms were ignored.

This isn't just about bad healthcare. It's about survival in our society. And this rings especially true for people with marginalized identities, those whose bodies haven't been treated with dignity in clinics, classrooms, relationships, or public spaces.

Maybe you've stopped mentioning certain symptoms because no one believed you last time. Maybe you've learned to stay vague so you won't get labeled. Maybe you dissociate during sex, skip meals without noticing, or push through pain until you crash. Maybe trauma made tuning out a necessary coping skill. Or maybe you've never once been asked, "What does your body need?" Or worse, maybe you've never even slowed down enough to ask yourself.

Survival mode isn't sustainable. You can't care for what you can't feel. And the longer we stay disconnected, the harder it becomes to name what's happening inside us. Until something explodes. A panic attack. A health crisis. Severe pain. A moment where you may realize, *I don't know what I feel right now or how I got here.*

Reconnection isn't instant. It's not clean or linear. But it *is* possible.

It starts with tiny moments. A pause. A breath. A check-in.

Part of healing from disconnection is reclaiming your body's language.

Learning how to understand it, and how to speak it.

## Start by Looking Back

Looking inward doesn't always mean meditating or journaling. Sometimes it means replaying the real-life moments when your body felt safe, and the ones when it didn't. That's where the clues live.

Before your next appointment, take a moment to reflect: When have you actually felt connected to your body? What helped you feel that way? Was it a particular environment? A person you trusted? A sense of calm or control?

What healthcare visits have gone better than others. Why? Was it the provider's tone? The way they explained things? Was it because you had a list prepared, or someone sitting beside you? Did you feel heard?

Now think about the opposite. What moments made you shut down? Did the room feel tense? Did you go blank or start second-guessing yourself? Did something in your body go quiet or flare?

These aren't just random memories. They're data. They show you what helps you feel steady, and what makes you disappear.

This is what listening inward looks like. It's not just about preparing your talking points for a provider. It's about knowing what your system needs to stay present. To stay connected. To stay *you*.

Sometimes that means choosing an appointment at a time of day when you're less anxious, or making sure you don't have to rush straight back to work. It might mean grounding yourself with music beforehand, or holding a smooth stone in your hand. It could mean asking to record the visit so you're not performing mental gymnastics trying to remember everything.

And afterward? Even so-called routine visits can leave you feeling exposed: physically, emotionally, or both. Maybe you finally said something out loud that you've been avoiding. Maybe you were dismissed. Or maybe it all went fine . . . and it still took a toll.

Give yourself a post-visit plan: a walk, a nap, an ice cream, a decompression call with someone who gets it. Your body doesn't clock out the moment the appointment ends. If you feel like you want it or need it, you deserve recovery in addition to preparation.

## Rebuilding Connection, One Check-In at a Time

You don't need to turn your body into a project or track every sensation in a color-coded spreadsheet. You just need to start paying attention.

You might begin with a simple daily check-in: *How does my body feel right now? Where do I feel tension, pain, comfort, ease?* Or once a week, do a gentle body scan from head to toe. Not to fix anything. Just to notice what's there.

You could jot down a few words, record a 30-second voice memo, or simply hold the awareness. Over time, you'll start to recognize patterns: *I always get headaches before my period. My energy dips after a certain meal. I clench my jaw when I'm around that person.*

That's information. And information is power. And the more information you have, the more connected you can be to yourself, and the more you can advocate for your own needs and experience.

You're not tuning in to overanalyze every moment. You're doing it to practice *noticing*. To gently disrupt the habit of dismissal that so many of us have been conditioned into.

## Create a Vocabulary for Your Experience

Part of advocating for yourself is learning how to describe what's going on. That doesn't necessarily mean using medical jargon. It means putting your experience into words that you can share with a provider who can understand and act accordingly.

Once you feel something, try to describe it. Try to identify it. Try to pinpoint it. Practice naming it out loud, even if it's just to yourself.

Instead of "I have pain," try the following:

- "It's a sharp pain on the left side that comes and goes."
- "It feels like a dull ache that radiates into my back."
- "It started two weeks ago and happens mostly at night."
- "It gets worse when I eat, better when I lie down."
- "It's worse during intercourse, especially in ___ position."

These aren't just details. They're clues. They can help you identify your symptoms, which can further shape your care.

And it's not just about pain. Track your energy. Your mood. Your digestion. Your sleep. If you menstruate, notice your bleeding patterns, premenstrual symptoms (PMS), and signs of ovulation. Even logging *felt off today, not sure why* is valid.

Over time, your body's language becomes clearer. You can understand it. You can vocalize it. You can live with a heightened awareness. A deeper connection to yourself. And then, you can ask for the care that you need.

## What's Normal for *You*?

One of the most disorienting questions patients ask is: "Is this normal?" But that question doesn't always help. Because normal is a range. *Your* normal is what matters. And getting in touch with your normal is how you can more easily identify the outliers.

Ask yourself these questions:

- *What does a typical month feel like for me?*
- *How does my body usually respond to stress?*
- *What's my baseline when it comes to sleep, digestion, libido, energy?*

Now ask these questions:

- *What feels different?*
- *How long has this change been happening?*
- *Is it better, worse, or staying the same?*
- *Is it interfering with my life?*

The better you know your own patterns, the easier it is to spot changes and speak up when something's off.

## What's Working and What's Not. Check-Ins That Change Everything

Tuning in doesn't always mean identifying a problem. Sometimes, it's about noticing what's working. What feels steady. What feels off. What you want to shift? Not just in your care, but in your *body*.

You can think of this as two separate check-ins: one inward, one outward. Both are equally important.

### Check In with Your Body

- What feels good in your body: physically or emotionally?
- What symptoms have improved, lessened, or stabilized?

- What's changed recently, for better or worse?
- What are the signals you've been ignoring or downplaying?

You might realize:

- *I have more energy in the mornings now.*
- *My periods are still heavy, but I'm managing them better.*
- *I'm clenching my jaw all day and didn't even notice.*
- *I haven't felt fully rested in months. And I'm ready to name that.*

These aren't just observations. They're intel. They tell you where you are right now. They help you notice your own rhythms, tolerances, and shifts. And they give you a foundation for the next check-in: your care.

### *Check In with Your Healthcare*

Now look at how you're being cared for, or not:

- What kinds of care have felt supportive, empowering, or affirming?
- What patterns in your past care have left you feeling small, dismissed, or unsafe?
- What are you ready to ask for that you haven't before?
- What are you done putting up with?

Maybe you're ready to say:

- "I'm done not sharing my true needs with my clinician."
- "I want pain meds offered, not just assumed optional."
- "I need a provider who uses affirming language about my body."
- "I want clearer follow-up, not another appointment where I leave confused."

This is about recognizing your own capacity and your right to expect more. It's okay to want to change your approach. To set new standards. To decide, *I've tried it that way. And now I'm doing it this way.*

You don't have to justify your needs. You just have to name them.

## When What You Need Feels Hard to Say

Bringing up sensitive topics is hard enough. Sexual pain. Mental health. Trauma. But when you add rushed appointments, a provider who doesn't make eye contact, a cold exam room, or a subtle shift in tone after you speak, it can feel impossible.

You might freeze. Or default to vague language. Or talk around the thing you really want to say. Not because you're unsure, but because it doesn't feel safe.

Maybe you've never said any of these things out loud. And it feels like ripping off a bandage but the moment has never felt right.

Maybe you've tried to bring it up before and got brushed off. Maybe you're scared of being labeled. Maybe you've been told you're exaggerating, overthinking, or "just anxious" by friends, family, or clinicians in the past. That kind of history doesn't disappear, it follows you into the room.

And so we protect ourselves. We make ourselves smaller. We prioritize comfort over honesty.

But the truth is: you don't owe anyone a polished version of your pain. You don't have to make it easy to hear in order for it to be valid.

You don't have to explain everything all at once. You can start small. You can pause. You can say, "This is hard for me to bring up."

Even that is brave. Even that matters.

Here's one way to ease into it: frame the issue as a quality-of-life concern or a pattern you've noticed. This helps providers take it seriously, while giving you a clear entry point.

- **For mental health:** "I've noticed some patterns I want to talk about."
- **For sexual health:** "This is affecting my quality of life, and I'd like to address it."

- **For trauma:** "There's some background I'd like you to know that may be relevant to my care."

Because every time you speak honestly about your body, your mind, your needs—you're taking back space in a system and a society that's long asked you to stay silent.

Silence doesn't serve you.

You're not being difficult. You're being honest. And honest is one of the bravest things you can be.

## It Doesn't Happen Overnight

Some days, you'll feel totally connected to your body. Other days, you'll want to check out. That's normal. Awareness isn't about perfection, it's about presence.

You're not broken. You're a whole person in a system and a society that often fragments people. Tuning in is about making space to hear what your body has been trying to tell you.

That might sound simple. But for many of us—especially those with a history of body shame, trauma, or dismissal—it's revolutionary.

## Build a Support Network That Gets It

You don't have to do this alone. Seek out people who talk about their bodies without shame. Talk about things. Name it with your friends. Don't let stigma or silence let you feel isolated. You'll find others who've had miscarriages, who've dealt with discharge, who've struggled with pain, or missed menses, or desire. In that shared truth, you'll feel less alone.

Explore books, podcasts, or online spaces that help you reconnect. Follow unapologetic leaders in the spaces that resonate. Build a care team that doesn't just treat your body but honors it.

You'll also get better at naming your own experience without apologizing for it. And then, you'll have and find providers who respect your body and your experience.

And when the system fails you, which it might, come back to this truth:

- Your symptoms are real.
- Your needs are valid.
- And your story and experience matters.

## The Bottom Line

Learning what you need doesn't require a medical degree. It requires curiosity, attention, and compassion.

You don't need to have all the answers. You just need to believe that your experience is worth listening to.

Because it is.

# Chapter 13

# Finding Care That Sees You

*Because the Right Provider Doesn't Just Treat Your Body. They Respect Your Whole Self*

Let's be real: not all providers are created equal. And not every clinician is equipped, or willing, to give you the kind of care you deserve. Sometimes it's just a mismatch in style. Other times, it's something deeper: bias, judgment, condescension, or outright harm. Whatever the reason, if you've ever walked out of a medical visit feeling unseen, misunderstood, or like you had to shrink yourself just to get through it, you're not alone. And it wasn't your fault.

This chapter isn't about blaming doctors. It's about how to find better ones. It's about getting clear on what you need, how to find it, and how to build care relationships that actually serve you. Not the other way around.

## Step 1: Define What You Need

Before you dive into Yelp reviews or start asking around, take a moment to get clear on your own needs. This isn't about being picky, it's about being prepared. Ask yourself these questions:

- Do I want someone who listens more than they talk?
- Is shared identity important: race, gender, orientation, faith, political affiliation?
- Do I need specific expertise (LGBTQ+ health, trauma, menopause, eating disorders, disability)?
- What communication style works for me? Direct and data-driven, or soft and exploratory?
- Do I prefer collaborative decision-making or a more guided, traditional approach?
- Are there values that matter? A reproductive justice lens, a body-positive philosophy, or cultural humility?
- Do I want a provider who can and will perform elective termination should I desire?

And just as important: name your dealbreakers. Think about past experiences that felt uncomfortable or unsafe. What kinds of language, assumptions, or behaviors are red flags for you? What's a hard no?

Finally, consider logistics:

- How far are you willing to travel for good care?
- Do you need evening or weekend hours?
- What insurance do you have, and what limitations might that place on your options?
- Is telehealth a viable part of your care strategy? Can you do a combination of in-person and telehealth?

Knowing this ahead of time will help you during your search. Once you're clear on what matters most to you, it's time to understand exactly *who* you might want on your care team.

## Step 2: Knowing Who's Who

Your reproductive healthcare is rarely a one-person job. The best care often comes from the right combination of people, a team whose skills complement each other, because it's unlikely that one provider can do it all. Before you can build that team, it helps to understand who does what, how their training differs, and where each one fits into your care.

When you start looking for care, it can feel like you're reading an alphabet soup of credentials: MD, DO, CNM, PA, NP. You may be wondering who actually does what. Here's a breakdown of who's who, what they do, and how they might fit into your team.

### *Obstetricians and Gynecologists (OB-GYN)*

OB-GYNs are physicians who specialize in obstetrics (pregnancy/birth) and gynecology (reproductive health across the lifespan). After four years of medical school, they complete a four-year residency that prepares them to manage everything from routine gynecologic care to high-risk pregnancies and complex surgeries. They are trained to diagnose, treat, and operate across a broad range of reproductive health needs, often being the provider who both delivers your baby and performs surgical procedures when needed.

### *Doctor of Medicine (MD) and Doctor of Osteopathic Medicine (DO)*

Both are fully licensed physicians. MDs (Doctors of Medicine) train in allopathic medicine; DOs (Doctors of Osteopathic Medicine) train in osteopathic medicine, which includes additional musculoskeletal training and a whole-person care philosophy. In practice, both can prescribe, operate, and deliver babies. The differences are more about philosophy and approach than scope of practice.

### Maternal-Fetal Medicine Specialist (MFM)

MFMs are OB-GYNs who complete an additional three years of fellowship focused on high-risk pregnancy care. They are the specialists you may see if you have a complicated pregnancy, such as multiples, preterm labor risk, fetal growth concerns, or preexisting medical conditions that make pregnancy riskier. MFMs offer advanced prenatal testing, manage complex maternal and fetal health issues, and often work closely with both you and your primary OB-GYN to coordinate a safe delivery plan.

### Reproductive Endocrinology and Infertility Specialist (REI)

REIs are OB-GYNs who go on to complete a three-year fellowship in reproductive endocrinology and infertility. They specialize in diagnosing and treating fertility challenges, hormonal disorders, recurrent pregnancy loss, and reproductive endocrine conditions like polycystic ovary syndrome (PCOS). They are trained in advanced fertility treatments such as in vitro fertilization (IVF), egg freezing, and embryo transfer, and often provide counseling and treatment plans tailored to your reproductive goals.

### Physician Associate / Physician Assistant (PA)

PAs are nationally certified, state-licensed clinicians trained in a master's-level medical model program (typically two to three years). The profession is shifting from *physician assistant* to *physician associate*, so you may see both terms used. They refer to the same role. In OB-GYN settings, they can perform exams, order and interpret tests, prescribe medications, and manage common gynecologic concerns. Because of their surgical training, PAs frequently first assist in procedures like C-sections, hysterectomies, and laparoscopies. Many patients value the additional time PAs can spend on education, follow-up, and shared decision-making in their care.

### Nurse Practitioner (NP)

NPs are registered nurses with graduate-level training (master's or doctorate) who can diagnose, treat, and prescribe. In OB-GYN care, women's health NPs and family NPs with gynecologic experience often manage routine visits, prenatal care, contraceptive counseling, and treatment of common concerns. Their nursing background often shapes a preventive, patient-centered approach that prioritizes health education alongside medical management.

### Certified Nurse Midwife (CNM)

CNMs are advanced practice registered nurses with graduate-level training in midwifery. They provide comprehensive reproductive, pregnancy, and postpartum care, can prescribe medications (including contraception), and, in many states, are the primary provider who manages the birth in hospitals, birth centers, or at home. Their care often blends medical expertise with a patient-centered approach, focusing on minimizing interventions when safe and supporting a low-intervention birth experience. CNMs work independently in some settings and in collaboration with physicians in others, ensuring seamless care if complications arise.

> PAs, NPs, and CNMs are often grouped together as advanced practice providers. In OB-GYN care, their roles often overlap: conducting routine visits, providing contraceptive counseling, managing prenatal care, and addressing problem-focused concerns. Because they may not carry the same surgical schedules or patient volume as physicians, they can often devote more time to conversation, education, and personalized care. For many patients, that extra space is the difference between leaving with unanswered questions and leaving with a clear, actionable plan. If you're not seeking surgical consultation but want a clinician who can listen, discuss your needs in depth, and partner with you in mapping out next steps, an advanced practice provider can be an excellent choice.

### Certified Professional Midwife (CPM)

CPMs are nationally certified midwives who are not nurses. Their training is midwifery-specific, often through accredited midwifery programs or structured apprenticeships, and focuses on providing care for low-risk pregnancies, births, and postpartum recovery in out-of-hospital settings. They are the primary provider who manages the birth in homes or freestanding birth centers, emphasizing physiologic birth, informed choice, and minimal intervention when safe. Unlike CNMs, CPMs generally cannot prescribe medications or serve as the clinical lead in hospital settings, though they are trained to recognize complications, provide emergency care, and coordinate timely transfers when needed. Their care model often incorporates cultural traditions, family involvement, and extended postpartum support.

### Doula

Doulas are trained, nonclinical support professionals who offer continuous emotional, physical, and informational support during pregnancy, birth, and postpartum. They do not provide medical care, but they play a vital role in advocacy, comfort, and helping you feel grounded and informed throughout your care. A doula's presence is associated with lower rates of intervention, higher satisfaction with birth experiences, and stronger feelings of support.

### Lactation Consultant (IBCLC)

International Board Certified Lactation Consultants (IBCLCs) are specialists in breastfeeding and chestfeeding who help with latch issues, milk supply, pumping, and feeding challenges. They may work in hospitals, clinics, or private practice, and provide both clinical guidance and emotional support during the often-challenging feeding journey. IBCLCs are trained to address both common concerns and complex situations, helping you meet your feeding goals.

### *Pelvic Floor Physical Therapist (PT)*

Pelvic floor PTs are licensed physical therapists with specialized training in pelvic health. They treat issues like pelvic pain, urinary or fecal incontinence, prolapse, and postpartum recovery concerns, as well as sexual dysfunction related to pelvic floor muscle health. They use targeted exercises, manual therapy, and education to restore function and improve quality of life, often working closely with OB-GYN teams.

### Genetic Counselor

Genetic counselors are healthcare professionals trained in medical genetics and counseling. They help you understand inherited conditions, assess personal or family health risks, and decide whether to pursue genetic testing. In reproductive care, they play a key role in prenatal screening, fertility planning, and navigating results in a supportive, nondirective way.

### *Ultrasonographer / Sonographer*

Ultrasonographers perform imaging studies such as pelvic or obstetric ultrasounds, using their training and expertise to capture the precise views your clinician needs to evaluate your reproductive and gynecologic health. While they are not the ones to give you an official diagnosis, they often have an extraordinary ability to recognize and document what's unfolding in real time, whether that's confirming an early pregnancy, assessing ovarian cysts, checking an intrauterine device's placement, or identifying fibroids. Many are true artists with the ultrasound probe, able to find the perfect angle, spot subtle details, and reveal that first glimpse of your baby or help visualize what's happening inside your body.

### *Psychologist / Talk Therapist*

Psychologists and other licensed therapists (such as clinical social workers or counselors) provide talk therapy to support mental and emotional health. In reproductive care, they play a critical role in helping patients navigate perinatal mood and anxiety disorders, grief after loss, sexual health concerns, and medical trauma. They are also key partners in trauma recovery, whether that's working through a difficult birth, a triggering medical experience, or past sexual trauma. Many use evidence-based approaches such as EMDR (eye movement desensitization and reprocessing) to help process and reframe these experiences so they have less emotional and physical impact in the future. While therapists cannot prescribe medication, they often work in close collaboration with psychiatrists, OB-GYNs, or midwives to ensure mental and emotional care is fully integrated into your treatment plan.

### *Psychiatrist*

Psychiatrists are medical doctors who specialize in mental health and can both prescribe medications and provide therapy. In reproductive healthcare, they can manage mental health conditions during pregnancy and postpartum, guide safe use of medications while breastfeeding, and support patients navigating mood or anxiety changes linked to hormonal shifts. Psychiatrists often collaborate with OB-GYNs, midwives, and therapists to integrate mental health into overall care.

### *Dietitian/Nutritionist (RD/RDN)*

Registered dietitians (RDs or RDNs) are credentialed experts in nutrition who can help manage conditions like PCOS, endometriosis, or gestational diabetes, and support fertility or postpartum recovery through nutrition. Not all "nutritionists" are licensed, so check credentials if you're seeking medical nutrition therapy.

## Step 3: Building a Team

Now that you know who's who, the next step is learning how they fit together, and how to choose the right person (or people) for the care you need right now.

Your primary care provider (PCP) is often at the center of your healthcare. Many PCPs provide basic gynecologic care like Pap smears, breast exams, STI testing, and contraception management. With the right PCP, you may not always need a specialist. Still, there will be times when you need someone with more advanced or focused training, and understanding these roles makes it easier to choose the right match for each part of your care.

Choosing a provider isn't about finding the "best" one in some universal sense. It's about finding the best one for you, in this moment. Scope and training matter: if you need surgery, advanced fertility treatment, or high-risk pregnancy care, you'll want a physician with that specific expertise. For routine care, contraceptive counseling, and preventive visits, a nurse practitioner, physician associate, or midwife may be a great choice. Philosophy and approach matter too. Some people want a hospital-based, highly medical model, while others prefer the time-rich, whole-person approach that midwives and advanced practice providers often offer.

Where care happens matters just as much as who provides it. Some services can be done safely in an outpatient clinic or birthing center, while others require a hospital setting. If you know you might need surgery, labor support, or hospital-based monitoring, choose someone with privileges at the hospital you prefer. If you're considering a birthing center or home birth, that comes with its own safety considerations and requires a certified professional midwife or certified nurse midwife who is trained in out-of-hospital birth and emergency management.

Continuity and comfort count too. Sometimes the best provider is the one you trust, who listens, and who makes you feel seen, even if their scope is narrower. And consider your specific needs: if you're postpartum and dealing with incontinence, a pelvic floor physical therapist is your go-to. Struggling with feeding? Call a lactation consultant. Planning pregnancy with a family history of certain conditions? A genetic counselor can help you map your options.

The best care rarely comes from a single person. It's built from the right combination of people. A team whose skills complement each other, because no one provider can do everything. Your needs will shift, and your team can shift with them. The real power comes from understanding who does what and choosing the person, or combination of people, who can give you the safest, most supportive, and most effective care for where you are right now.

## Step 4: Smart Searching Strategies

When you're ready to look, start within your network. Ask friends who share your values or lived experience. Reach out to organizations you respect, healthcare providers you like, therapists, local reproductive justice groups, LGBTQ+ centers, or support groups.

If you're turning to the internet, use specific search terms. You can also explore specialized directories. This step can take time. But remember, you're interviewing them, not the other way around. And always check your insurance coverage before booking; knowing what's in-network can make a big difference in cost.

## Step 5: Centering Identity and Experience in Your Search

The right provider isn't just clinically skilled, they see you as a whole person. That means your care is shaped not only by their medical expertise but also by their ability to understand and respect the identity and experiences you bring into the room.

This might be about finding someone who shares your background, or about finding someone who doesn't but who has done the work to honor it. It might be about seeking a provider who understands the nuances of your gender, sexuality, race, disability, faith, or health history. Or it might be about choosing someone whose values align with yours, especially when it comes to reproductive rights, bodily autonomy, and the kind of care you believe you deserve.

Your identity and your lived experience aren't side notes in your medical chart, they're central to how you'll experience care, how safe you'll feel, and how likely you are to get what you need without feeling dismissed or misunderstood. Knowing this up front gives you permission to prioritize finding a provider who not only *can* care for you but who also will care for you in a way that feels affirming, respectful, and aligned.

### *If You're Queer*

Look for providers who do more than wave a Pride flag. You deserve someone trained in queer health. Someone who understands sexual health across diverse relationships, is fluent in inclusive language, and is mindful of the ways stigma and bias can show up in the exam room. They should also be comfortable discussing same-sex family planning options, including donor sperm, reciprocal IVF, and adoption so your care supports your goals for building a family. Bonus if their forms, policies, and staff reflect that same fluency.

### *If You're Trans*

Seek out providers with real experience in gender-affirming care, including hormone therapy, post-surgical care, and the ways gender-affirming treatment can interact with reproductive health. They should be prepared to discuss fertility preservation and family-building options in ways that affirm your gender and align with your goals. Their language, forms, and physical space should signal safety, not just tolerance.

### If You're a Patient of Color

Culturally responsive care isn't just a buzzword, it's essential. That might mean working with a BIPOC provider, or with someone who's done the work to understand racial bias and health disparities. You shouldn't have to teach your provider how to treat you with dignity.

### If You Have a History of Trauma

Find a trauma-informed provider who understands how past traumatic experiences, medical, sexual, or otherwise, can affect comfort in the exam room. Ask if they can modify procedures, use grounding techniques, or allow a support person to be present.

### If You're Disabled

Ask up front about accessibility: adjustable exam tables, visual or communication aids, flexible scheduling. More important, look for someone who respects your autonomy and doesn't see your disability as the whole story.

### If You Have Chronic Illness or Multiple Specialists

Choose a provider who communicates well with your broader care team. Coordination is key, especially if you're managing medications or conditions that affect reproductive health.

### If You Have Complex Medical Care or History

Look for someone with the same or compatible electronic medical record system so they can review notes, see labs, and ensure your care is consistent across settings.

### If You're Navigating Menopause or Perimenopause

Seek a provider who has up-to-date training in menopausal care and can address hormonal and nonhormonal options, sexual health, and mental health during this transition. Many clinicians receive little formal education in this stage, so it's worth asking directly about their experience.

### *If Your Faith Guides Your Choices*

Your spirituality might shape how you approach birth control, fertility, pregnancy, or abortion. That's valid. Ask if the provider is comfortable discussing religious values and how they'll factor into your care. Affirming care should meet you where you are, including in your beliefs.

### *If Progressive Values Matter to You*

You may want a provider who doesn't just offer abortion care, but believes in it. Someone who supports trans rights, reproductive justice, and bodily autonomy out loud. That kind of alignment can be grounding, especially in a time when reproductive rights are under attack.

### *If You're an Immigrant or Undocumented*

Look for clinics that understand immigrant-specific barriers, such as language access, confidentiality concerns, and insurance or payment flexibility. Some have patient advocates who can help you navigate care without putting your safety at risk.

### *If You Live in a Rural Area*

Your options may be shaped by geography. In rural areas, telehealth can expand access, especially for contraception, hormone management, and counseling. Ask about virtual care, satellite clinics, or coordinated visits that let you combine multiple services in one trip.

## Step 6: Read the Signs (Online and Off)

Once you've got a few names, do your research. Don't just glance at star ratings. Dig into the reviews and pay attention to the emotional tone. Look for signs that the provider listens, makes patients feel comfortable, doesn't rush, respects pronouns, validates concerns, and takes time to explain things clearly. Just as important, watch for the red flags that tell you this might not be the right fit: comments about feeling rushed, not being taken seriously, being judged for weight, having identity misunderstood, or pain dismissed. The language patients use in reviews can tell you as much about the provider as their credentials ever will.

A provider's online presence also says a lot. You want to see yourself reflected there. Does it center the things that matter to you? Is their website inclusive? Are their forms gender-inclusive? Do they show diverse staff? Have they done any public-facing education or advocacy?

These things aren't guarantees, but they're signals.

## Step 7: Use the Phone Call as a Screen

Before you even walk into the exam room, you can learn a lot from the way a clinic answers the phone. When you call to schedule, ask questions that go beyond the standard script. Inquire whether providers have experience with LGBTQ+ or trans patients, if intake forms are gender-inclusive, and how the clinic approaches trauma-informed care. Ask if they have accessible equipment for larger bodies or patients with disabilities, and where it's safe and legal to do so, how the provider approaches reproductive autonomy and abortion. Keep in mind that in some states, staff may not feel comfortable or be permitted to answer this directly due to fear of retaliation. If faith or political values play a role in your care preferences, you can also ask whether the provider is open to discussing those topics in a respectful way.

Pay attention to the answers but also the tone. Does the person seem annoyed you're asking? Or are they affirming, helpful, and curious? And, yes, the front desk isn't the provider, but the vibe still matters. How the clinic operates tells you a lot about the kind of care you can expect once you walk through the door.

## Step 8: The Appointment Gut Check

Your first visit is your test drive. Pay attention not just to what the provider says but also to how they make you feel. Green flags include using your correct name and pronouns, asking about your goals and preferences, explaining what they're doing before touching you, checking in during the exam, respecting your questions without brushing them off, asking if you feel safe or need accommodations, and inviting your feedback or corrections. Red flags include making assumptions about your gender, sexuality, lifestyle, or politics; showing discomfort when you ask for clarification; dismissing pain or concerns; shaming you for past choices; or ignoring your requests for boundaries.

Keep in mind, during a first visit you absolutely do not have to have a pelvic exam, or any physical exam, if you don't want to. You can use that initial appointment as a meet-and-greet, a conversation, or a planning session to decide whether this is someone you want on your care team. If you'd prefer to skip an exam, you can say, "I'd like to focus on talking through my history and questions today and save the physical exam for a later visit."

Sure, it's frustrating to leave if you've taken the time to find the right office, make the appointment, and maybe take time off work to be there. But if it doesn't feel good or feel right, remember: you're the boss of your own healthcare. You set the boundaries. You decide who gets to be on your team.

## Step 9: Working Around Geography

Not everyone has a wealth of options nearby. If you live in a rural area, a region hostile to reproductive rights, or a place with limited provider diversity, it can feel like good care just isn't available. But telehealth has changed the game.

Virtual appointments can cover a wide range of needs: birth control consults, STI treatment, gender-affirming hormone therapy, menopausal care, medication abortion, and general reproductive counseling. You can also use telehealth for second opinions, follow-ups, or navigating complex choices with someone who gets it.

Many patients create a hybrid model that works for their reality: they use local clinics or urgent care for labs and physical exams, lean on telehealth for ongoing support, and travel occasionally to see a trusted specialist. It's not always perfect, but it can be powerful. Especially when it means you get affirming care, even if it's not just down the street. There's no one-size-fits-all solution. What matters is that the setup supports you.

## Step 10: If It's Not Working, Keep Looking

A provider can be kind and still not be the right fit for you. They can be brilliant on paper and still miss the mark in practice. If you leave appointment after appointment feeling drained, small, or more confused than when you walked in, it's worth reevaluating.

You have full permission to keep searching. To switch providers, cancel your next visit, or even walk out mid-appointment if something feels wrong. This isn't about being picky; it's about protecting your health and your peace of mind. Your standards don't make you difficult, they make you someone who knows their worth and refuses to settle for care that doesn't meet it.

## The Bottom Line

Finding the right reproductive healthcare provider is part strategy, part intuition, and part persistence. You may not get it right the first time. But you deserve to keep trying until it clicks. Because the right provider doesn't just examine you. They see you.

They respect your body and your story. Your identity and your autonomy. Your goals and your boundaries. They make space for your full self in the exam room and in your care team.

## Chapter 14

# How to Get Ready, Speak Up, and Handle What Comes

*Speaking Up Is Power; Knowing What to Do When You're Dismissed Is Protection*

Think about this: there's a whole trend online of women admitting they'd rather live with a bad manicure than speak up at the nail salon. They'll pick out a color, watch the technician start painting, and instantly know it's not what they wanted. Maybe the shade looks different under the lights. Maybe the shape feels wrong. But even as that sinking feeling hits, *this isn't right*, the thought of saying something feels harder than swallowing the discomfort. So they sit quietly, hand over their money, and spend weeks staring at nails they hate, all because they didn't want to make things "awkward."

It seems trivial. It's just nail polish, right? But what's happening in that chair isn't really about the nails. It's about the clash between discomfort and confrontation. For many of us, the fear of being seen as demanding or ungrateful feels so unbearable that we'd rather carry dissatisfaction for weeks than risk a 30-second correction.

Now translate that same instinct into a medical setting. Only here, it's not about the color of your nails. It's the care plan for your body. Silence at the salon leaves you annoyed every time you look at your hands. Silence in the exam room can leave you living with months of untreated bleeding, pain that keeps you from work, or unanswered questions about your fertility or your future. The same reflex that keeps you quiet in the chair—*don't make it awkward, don't be difficult*—is the one that lets a provider move past your concerns without ever addressing them.

And the system banks on that silence. It survives on patients who don't push back, who don't correct, who don't say, "This isn't working for me." Speaking up at the nail salon might save you a week of annoyance. Speaking up in the exam room could change the course of your care, or even save your life.

We'd all love to believe we can just show up to a doctor's appointment, describe what's going on, and walk out with a clear plan. But most of us know that's rarely how it goes. You wait. You undress. You try to remember the right words. There's never enough time. The visit moves fast, the explanations feel thin, and before you know it, it's over. And somehow, you still don't have answers.

This chapter isn't here to repeat what you already know about short visits or broken systems. It's here to give you a strategy. To reclaim your voice. Not just to speak, but to ask. To interrupt. To clarify. Because those moments, the ones where you ask a better question or pause a conversation that's going sideways, those are where your power lives.

## The Day Before: Emotional and Practical Prep

A good visit starts before you ever step into the room. A day or two before, pause and check in with yourself:

- *What's really bothering me?*
- *What do I want to walk out with?*

- *What would make this visit feel successful?*

Turn those answers into a simple hierarchy:

- **Primary issue:** The one thing that must get addressed
- **Main goal:** The action you want to come out of that discussion
- **Bonus goal:** A secondary concern, only if time allows

Write it down. Bring it with you. This isn't overkill. It's a way of keeping the visit focused on what matters most to you.

Next, shape your "symptom story" into three parts:

- **The what:** A clear description of the problem
- **The impact:** How it affects your daily life
- **The timeline:** When it started and how it has changed

Pair that with any evidence you've got. Tracking app screenshots, photos, a list of medications you've tried. And practice a one-liner to ground you when nerves hit: "I'm here because my periods have become unbearable and I need help figuring out why."

Before you leave the house, pack the basics: your list of goals, insurance card and ID, medication list, pharmacy info, notebook, phone, and, if you'd like, a support person. Preparation doesn't make you pushy. It makes you ready.

## In the Room: Asking the Right Questions

Once you're face-to-face, the difference often comes down to the questions you ask. When a provider says, "Watch and wait," try asking these questions:

- *"What specifically should I be watching for?"*
- *"If it gets worse, what's our next step?"*
- *"Can we make a plan now for what happens if nothing changes?"*

When they order tests:

- *"What are we looking for?"*
- *"What happens if it's normal? What if it's not?"*

When they give a diagnosis:

- "What does this mean for my daily life?"
- "How will we know if this treatment is working?"
- "If this were your sister, what would you tell her?"

These aren't confrontational. They're clarifying. And they shift you from passive patient to informed partner.

## When the System Pushes Back

Sometimes, even when you ask all the right questions, you'll hear no. Often that wall isn't your provider's personal opinion, it's the guidelines they're bound by. Specialty societies like American College of Obstetricians and Gynecologists or the US Preventive Services Task Force set recommendations on when a test or treatment is "indicated." In theory, they're minimum standards. In practice, they can act like hard limits.

That's why you might request a screening and hear, "It's not indicated." Insurance companies, hospital administrators, and liability concerns all reinforce those walls.

But knowing this lets you probe differently:

- "What would it take for this to be considered indicated in my case?"
- "Is there a way to document my request so insurance might cover it?"
- "What are the risks, for you or me, if we go outside the guideline?"

The block isn't that your voice wasn't loud enough. It's that the system is wired to keep boundaries tight. Understanding that helps you decide when to push, when to pivot, and when to ask for another path.

## If Things Go South: Your Emergency Playbook

And sometimes, despite it all, the visit still goes bad. You feel ignored, talked over, or pressured. That's when it helps to have reset lines ready if feeling:

- **Dismissed:** "I understand this might be common, but it's not normal for me. What else can we try?"
- **Judged:** "I'm feeling shamed right now, and that's not helping. Can we refocus on my care?"
- **Interrupted:** "Let me finish my thought, then I'd love to hear your perspective."
- **Told to wait it out:** "I'm not comfortable with that approach. Can we talk about alternatives?"

These aren't about being difficult. They're about drawing the line back to your care.

## When Speaking Up Still Isn't Enough

I want to pause here and be honest about something important. These strategies—questions, scripts, reset lines—can be powerful tools. They can change the tone of a visit. They can help you get the care you deserve.

But here's the truth: they don't always work. Not because you didn't use them right, or because you weren't brave enough. I've heard too many stories of patients being berated, dismissed, or even "fired" from a practice simply for advocating for themselves. That is not okay. And it is not your fault.

So if you try a script and it backfires, please hear me: you didn't do it wrong. You did the best you could inside a broken system. The burden should not fall on you alone to fix it. Providers and institutions need to change, too.

And sometimes, things cross a line. If your provider refuses to answer your questions, dismisses your symptoms without an exam, shames your identity or body, crosses physical boundaries, or pressures you into treatments you're not ready for, it may be time to consider leaving. Walking away isn't dramatic, it's protective.

It's not always the first option, but it should always be on the table when care no longer feels safe or respectful. You have the right to pause or stop an exam, ask for a chaperone, request a different provider, leave mid-visit, or simply say no. These are your rights. Full stop.

Until the system changes, all you can do is protect your peace, know your rights, and remember: your voice matters. And so does your exit.

## When the Visit Goes Well

Not every visit feels like a fight. Some remind you why you keep showing up: because care done well can feel steady, respectful, even healing. When that happens, take note. These moments matter, not just for you, but for the relationship you're building.

Trust grows in layers. It builds when a provider explains things clearly instead of rushing. When they pause to check in. When they invite your perspective into the plan instead of treating your words as background noise.

Trust doesn't erase the hard visits that came before. But it does create a blueprint for what care can look like when it's working. Over time, those patterns matter. They show your nervous system it's possible to walk into a visit without every guard raised, every defense on high alert. That's not blind faith, it's earned confidence.

Name those moments out loud: "I really appreciated how you explained that" or "You made me feel heard today." It may feel small, but to your provider it's huge. It tells them clearly, "This worked; please keep doing it."

As a clinician, I can tell you firsthand: it means the world. The ones who make the effort to listen are often running late, getting chastised by their supervisors, and swimming against a system that punishes them for slowing down. Your acknowledgment, whether in the room or in a thank-you note, isn't just kindness. It's fuel. It's what makes the effort feel worthwhile, and what reminds them why they chose this work in the first place.

And just as a negative review can hold bad care accountable, a positive one can be just as powerful. It not only boosts morale for providers who are fighting to do right by their patients. It also helps other patients find them. A thoughtful review that says, "I felt heard," "They explained things clearly," or "I never felt rushed," can be a beacon for someone scrolling through options, desperate to know where they'll be treated with respect. In a system where so much energy goes into calling out harm, shining a light on what good care looks like is a form of advocacy, too.

## After a Bad Visit: Recovery Protocol

A hard visit doesn't end when you walk out the door. It follows you home. In your chest, in your jaw, in the loop of replaying every word. The feelings pile up: resentment that you weren't heard, anger at being dismissed, frustration with a system that wastes your time, and sometimes even shame for not speaking up the way you wish you had. You start second-guessing yourself: *Did I push too hard? Not hard enough? Should I have said something different?*

If you're leaving a visit feeling frustrated, dismissed, angry, or resentful, remember: it is not your fault. These feelings aren't proof you failed; they're proof the system did. Here are some tools to help you move through them:

- **Ground.** Notice where the visit lives in your body. Tight shoulders, a pit in your stomach, a racing mind. Naming it helps loosen its grip.
- **Connect.** Say it out loud to someone you trust: a friend, a therapist, even a group chat. Speaking the words restores perspective.

- **Reflect.** Write down what happened and, just as important, what you wish had happened. This isn't dwelling. It's drafting your blueprint for next time.
- **Reframe.** Remind yourself: a bad visit says more about the system than it does about you. It's data, not a verdict on your worth.
- **Plan.** Once the emotions have eased, start thinking about what comes next. Do you want to follow up, clarify, seek a second opinion, or walk away altogether? Naming your next step keeps you moving forward instead of stuck in the bad experience.

When you've steadied yourself, you can move from emotional recovery into practical recovery:

**Step 1: Document everything.** Jot down what happened. What was said, what felt off, what wasn't addressed, and how you felt in the moment. Getting it out of your head and onto paper (or into your Notes app) gives you something solid to reference later.

**Step 2: Check the visit notes.** Log into your patient portal. Read what they documented. Screenshot anything that doesn't match your memory or experience. Make sure you have access to any lab values or tests ordered should you wish to reference them later.

**Step 3: Take the next step.** Whatever you decided in your plan, now is the time to put it into motion. Whether that's sending a follow-up message, scheduling another visit, or beginning the process of finding a new provider.

**Step 4: Report, if needed.** If a line was crossed—whether through discrimination, boundary violations, or serious lapses in care—you have every right to speak up. Start with the practice manager or patient advocate, and escalate if necessary. A public review can also protect other patients, but keep it thoughtful, not retaliatory.

Bad care leaves marks, but it doesn't define you. Processing the fallout is part of protecting your energy, and part of building the confidence to walk back in, on your terms.

## Your Care, Your Terms

You deserve care that makes you feel respected, not rushed. Care that builds plans with you, not for you.

And if you don't get that? You deserve to walk away. Your job isn't to be agreeable. It's to be honest. To name what isn't working. To take your trust somewhere it will be honored.

The next time you walk into an exam room, don't go in empty-handed. Bring your questions, your scripts, your strategies. Bring the lived knowledge that your experience matters. That doesn't make you "difficult." It makes you prepared.

And prepared patients change what care feels like, one room at a time.

# Chapter 15

# Asking for Pain Management

*You Shouldn't Have to Suffer Through It, but You Do Need to Ask Ahead of Time*

There's a long, ugly history in medicine of not believing women when we say something hurts. It shows up in emergency rooms. It shows up in primary care. And it absolutely shows up in reproductive healthcare, where we're expected to endure procedures on the most sensitive parts of our bodies with little more than a deep breath and a "just try to relax."

Too many people walk into an appointment thinking they'll just push through. That it can't be that bad. That they're supposed to handle it. And too many walk out stunned—by how much it hurt, how little support they got, and how casually that pain was brushed off.

And for Black, brown, disabled, and LGBTQ+ patients, pain dismissal is even more common, rooted in long-standing biases that still shape whose pain is believed.

It doesn't have to be this way.

## The Physiology of Pain

One reason reproductive pain is so often dismissed is because many providers were trained to see it as minor. Something patients should be able to "tolerate." But the truth is, pain in the cervix and uterus is different from pain in other parts of the body, and there are real physiologic reasons why it can feel so intense.

The cervix and uterus have a dense network of nerves, and many of those nerves connect to the vagus nerve, which controls automatic responses like heart rate and blood pressure. When those nerves are triggered, say, during an intrauterine device (IUD) insertion, biopsy, or dilation, the uterus can cramp forcefully, and the body can sometimes respond with dizziness, sweating, nausea, or even fainting (a vagal response). None of this is "in your head." It's a normal physiologic reaction to stimulation in one of the most sensitive areas of the body.

Another reason the pain feels overwhelming is because of how the uterus contracts. Uterine cramping isn't just a twinge. It's muscle squeezing hard to push something out or resist something coming in. If you've ever had severe period cramps, you know how consuming that kind of pain can be. Procedures on the cervix or uterus tap directly into that same system, often more intensely and without warning.

And here's something important: pain is always subjective. That means your pain is real no matter how anyone else describes theirs. One person might experience an IUD insertion as uncomfortable but tolerable. Another might find it excruciating. Both are true. What matters isn't whether your pain matches a provider's expectations. It's what you feel.

## Prompting the Conversation

Your provider may not bring up pain management. Not because they don't care, but because most were trained to see these procedures as quick, routine, no big deal. Many clinicians have never been taught in-office pain protocols, and most have never experienced these procedures themselves. It's easy to underestimate something you've only ever performed, not endured.

That's why phrases like "You'll feel a little pinch" or "Just a small cramp" are so common. They're meant to help patients feel calm. But reassurance without honesty can backfire. When the pain is far worse than advertised, patients don't just feel hurt, they feel blindsided, dismissed, and even betrayed. What was meant to soothe ends up deepening mistrust.

This is why asking about pain management, *and doing it in advance*, is essential. Some options require planning, like prescribing medication ahead of time. And for many procedures—like IUD insertions, colposcopies, endometrial biopsies, cervical dilations, uterine aspirations, or anything involving the cervix or uterus—pain is real.

If you have a history of anxiety, sexual trauma, chronic pelvic pain, or simply know your body is sensitive, that pain can be even more intense. Planning isn't a luxury. It's a necessity.

Even pain from something as everyday as hemorrhoids or anal fissures is often brushed off instead of treated like the real, disruptive problem it is. The same goes for ovarian cysts. Just because a cyst looks small on ultrasound doesn't mean the pain should be minimized. Period cramps that flatten someone for days, pelvic floor muscle spasms, pain during sex, and even recovery pain after childbirth are all too often waved away as if they're inevitable, so the pain goes ignored and unsupported.

And sometimes, pain isn't the only concern. If you have vasovagal syncope, a physical response where your body can faint or go lightheaded during medical procedures, it's important to plan for that, too. This isn't about fear or emotion. It's a well-documented physiologic reflex that can happen with blood draws, Pap smears, IUD insertions, or cervical exams. If you've fainted during a medical visit before, your provider needs to know. Ask what they can do to support you, and consider bringing someone with you if that feels safer.

In 2025, clinical guidelines finally caught up to what patients have been saying for decades: gynecologic procedures can be painful, and pain management should be offered up front, not only if someone begs for it. These guidelines didn't create a new truth—they finally acknowledged an old one: patients were right about pain all along. The updated standards emphasize shared decision-making, advance preparation, and individualized care. Not one-size-fits-all assumptions.

It's a step forward. But guidelines doesn't rewrite clinical practice overnight. And for now, the burden too often still falls on patients to bring it up first.

## What's Actually Available: A Menu of Pain Management Options

Every body is different, and every procedure lands differently. There's no one-size-fits-all answer, which is why the best approach is a plan made with you, not for you. Here are some of the options worth asking about:

- **Over-the-counter pain relievers (ibuprofen or naproxen).** These can help with cramping *after* certain procedures, like an endometrial biopsy, but they don't do much for pain *during* something like an IUD insertion. Still, they're often recommended as a baseline.
- **Local anesthetics (lidocaine gel, spray, or a paracervical block).** These are some of the most effective options for reducing pain during procedures involving the cervix or uterus, like IUDs, colposcopies, biopsies, or aspirations. If you don't hear them offered, bring them up directly. These numbing options are safe, effective, and recommended in updated guidelines—patients shouldn't have to advocate this hard for something so basic.
- **Nitrous oxide ("laughing gas").** Sometimes available in outpatient settings, nitrous oxide can help reduce both pain and anxiety during procedures. Not every clinic has it, but if it's offered, it can be a great option for people who want support without full sedation.

- **Sedation, when indicated.** For some procedures, especially if you've had difficult past experiences, sedation may be an option. This requires planning ahead, often a driver, and not every setting can provide it, but it's worth asking if you feel you'll need deeper support.
- **Anti-anxiety medication (a one-time dose).** This doesn't take away pain, but it can help calm your body's stress response if anxiety is a big piece of the experience. You'll need to ask ahead of time, since it requires a prescription and you'll likely need a driver, too.
- **Support for fainting (vasovagal syncope).** If you've fainted with medical procedures before, tell your provider. They may adjust positioning, monitor you more closely, or recommend you bring someone with you. Planning for this isn't overreacting, it's being safe.
- **Non-drug comfort measures.** Heat packs, breathing strategies, distraction (music, conversation), or simply being given extra time. These won't erase pain, but they can make the overall experience more manageable.
- **The right to pause.** This one isn't in any guideline, but it matters: you have the right to ask your provider to stop or take a break if the pain becomes too much.

## How to Ask About Pain Management

Some clinics simply aren't set up with these tools yet, not necessarily because they don't care, but because they haven't updated their protocols or training. That's why asking ahead of time matters. And far too often, pain management isn't even mentioned unless you bring it up first. That doesn't mean you can't ask. In fact, naming it directly can change the entire tone of the visit. Here's what that might sound like in real life:

- "I'm really nervous about how painful this might be. What are my options for pain management?"

- "Can I take ibuprofen or naproxen beforehand?" (For some procedures, like an endometrial biopsy, it may help with cramping afterward. For IUDs, though, studies show it doesn't do much during the insertion itself, so it's worth asking what else they can offer.)
- "Do you offer numbing options like lidocaine gel, spray, or a paracervical block?" (These are some of the most effective ways to reduce pain during procedures like IUDs, biopsies, or aspirations. They should be on the table.)
- "Can I take something right before the appointment to help with anxiety? I don't need it for daily use, just to get through the procedure." (Some providers will prescribe a one-time anti-anxiety medication. It won't take the pain away, but it can make the experience more manageable if anxiety is a big part of it for you.)
- "I've fainted during procedures before. How can we plan for that this time?"
- "I've had a hard time with procedures like this in the past, and I want to make sure we plan for that."
- "Will I be okay to go back to work afterward, or should I plan for downtime?" (Even if they say you'll be fine, trust your own body and what you know about how you tend to respond.)
- "If this ends up being too uncomfortable, I want to know we can pause or stop."

None of these questions make you difficult. They make you prepared. They shift the conversation from "just get through it" to "let's make a plan." And the truth is, a plan changes everything: it gives you more control, more options, and more confidence walking into the room.

## Red Flags: When Pain Isn't Taken Seriously

Not every provider is ready for this conversation. Some may get defensive or act like you're overreacting. That's not your fault—and it's not a reason to stay silent.

Watch for these warning signs:

- They brush off your concerns with "It won't be that bad" or "Most people handle it fine."
- They refuse to discuss pain management at all.
- They insist there are "no options" or only suggest over-the-counter meds without explanation.
- They shame you for asking, implying you're being dramatic, weak, or difficult.
- They act impatient or irritated when you bring up past experiences or fears.
- They move ahead with a procedure after you've asked to pause or stop.

Pain isn't just physical, it's emotional. And when it's ignored or dismissed, the damage lasts long after the procedure is over. You are always allowed to pause an exam. To ask for a chaperone. To say, "I'm not comfortable with this." You can stop the visit. You can ask for a different provider. You can leave. And you can come back another day, with a better plan and someone by your side.

If your provider won't even engage in a conversation about pain, that's not your failure. It's a signal the care itself isn't respecting you.

## When Pain Goes Viral

The reason videos about IUD pain rack up millions of views isn't because people love watching suffering. It's because those shaky, handheld clips finally break the silence medicine has kept for too long. A wobbly phone camera in a clinic chair captures what most textbooks, and even most providers, leave out: the very real pain of procedures done on the cervix and uterus.

Scroll through the comments and you'll see the same chorus again and again: "I thought I was weak." "This happened to me too." "Why didn't anyone warn me?"

What spreads isn't just fear. It's validation. Patients who were brushed off in real time suddenly see their own experiences reflected back, magnified, and believed by thousands of strangers. In a culture where women and gender-diverse patients have long been told to grit their teeth, TikTok is rewriting the script in real time. Instead of providers deciding what counts as pain, patients hold the camera. Instead of isolated stories whispered one-on-one, testimony is collective.

These videos matter because they show the cost of underestimating pain. A single viral post can ripple across entire communities. Convincing someone to skip the birth control they wanted, or to delay a needed procedure. Providers sometimes roll their eyes and say, "Social media is scaring people." But the truth is the opposite. Patients aren't scared because of TikTok. They're scared because no one warned them. TikTok just said the quiet part out loud.

That's the cultural shift: pain isn't invisible anymore. It's documented. It's amplified. And it's shared so widely that the medical system no longer gets the last word. The only question is whether healthcare will catch up—by listening, validating, and offering pain management up front—before the gap between patients' reality and providers' assumptions grows even wider.

And if providers choose to listen? Then those same viral videos stop being warnings and start becoming catalysts. They become proof points that patients were right all along. A push for medicine to finally meet people where they are. Social media has already changed the conversation. Now healthcare has the chance to change the care.

## Breaking the Cycle of Pain and Silence

The stories people share online don't just raise awareness, they leave an imprint. Seeing someone faint during an IUD insertion, or remembering your own biopsy that left you shaken, can make the idea of another appointment feel unbearable. That's the ripple effect of pain left unaddressed: it doesn't stop when the procedure ends. It lingers, and it shapes whether people come back.

But this is exactly where the cycle can break. Avoiding care isn't the answer, better care is. And better care starts with one simple shift: treating pain as something worth preventing, not just enduring. Planning for pain before it happens changes everything.

When you ask about pain management ahead of time, you're not just protecting yourself for this visit, you're reshaping what care is allowed to look like. Every time a patient speaks up, it pushes back on the old assumption that pain is just part of the deal. It reminds providers, and it reminds all of us, that comfort isn't a luxury. It's the baseline.

Because the truth is, one rough IUD, one biopsy brushed off as "just a pinch," that can be enough to scare someone away from care for years. Asking early, planning ahead, and knowing you deserve better is how you stop that from happening to you. And collectively, it's how we change what patients expect and what providers prepare for.

## Naming the Pain

It's not just that we lack solutions for pain. Too often, we avoid even admitting how much it can hurt. When pain is downplayed or skipped over entirely, what lingers isn't only the pain itself but the shock of feeling unprepared.

This shows up especially in self-managed abortion care. The instructions are almost always the same: take some ibuprofen, grab a heating pad, try to rest. Those things help, but they aren't magic. Patients are often told it will feel like a heavy, crampy period. But in reality, it can be far worse for some. When the pain rises above what they were led to expect, many start to worry something is wrong, because no one warned them it might feel like this. Support hotlines hear from patients all the time who are caught off guard, calling in panicked because the reality is so different from what they were told. Time and time again, the problem isn't just the pain itself, it's the fear created when the truth gets downplayed.

What patients often need most in those moments isn't a miracle fix, it's validation. To hear "Yes, this can hurt. Yes, you're doing it right. Yes, you will get through it." Pain is not a sign of failure, and it doesn't always mean something is wrong. I wish there were a way to take it all away. Sometimes, pain is simply part of the process.

Some of the strategies in this chapter, like antianxiety medications, numbing agents, or pre-procedure pain relief, can absolutely make a difference. But most won't erase pain completely. And that matters, because patients deserve the full truth. You shouldn't be minimized into believing it won't hurt, and you shouldn't be dismissed if you ask for relief. The honest answer is both/and. Yes, there are ways to manage pain. And yes, sometimes it will still really hurt.

Naming the pain isn't about scaring people, it's about preparing them. Sometimes the most radical form of pain management is simply telling the truth.

## What Better Care Looks Like

When pain is taken seriously, it changes everything. You feel safer. More in control. Less ashamed. You leave the appointment as a partner in your care. Not a passive body on a table.

Ask early. Ask clearly. Expect answers that treat you like a person. Your comfort isn't an afterthought. It's part of the care.

And no, you're not asking for too much. You're asking for what you deserve. In fact, you're asking for what's finally being recognized as the standard. Those 2025 guidelines say it plainly: pain management should be offered, planned for, and treated as essential, not optional. That shift is a turning point, proof that what patients have been saying for decades was right all along.

Because this isn't just about medicine. It's about a culture that has long treated women's pain as an inconvenience, our needs as negotiable, and our discomfort as something to be endured quietly. Better care means breaking that pattern. It means finally believing people when they say they hurt, and building a system where comfort is not a bonus, but the baseline.

# Chapter 16

# Care Beyond the Exam Room

*Self-Care Isn't Separate from Healthcare, It's Part of It*

Advocating for your own needs takes energy. Walking into exam rooms prepared, asking the right questions, pushing back against dismissal, navigating insurance, demanding pain management. It's necessary work, but it can leave you wrung out. And the truth is, the hard part doesn't always end when the appointment does. Sometimes it's what comes after: replaying what was said, sitting with what wasn't addressed, or carrying the weight of it all on your own.

This chapter is about what happens in those spaces in between. It's about letting yourself lean on others instead of holding everything alone. It's about finding ways to reclaim your body and restore your energy when the system leaves you drained. And it's about protecting yourself. Keeping your own record, knowing your rights, and refusing to let a broken system define your care.

Because care doesn't end at the exam room door. How you tend to yourself afterward is part of the care you deserve.

## Seeking Support

Advocacy can feel like a solo act. You're the one sitting on the table, fielding the questions, fighting to be heard. But care doesn't have to be carried alone. Support is part of the picture too, not as a luxury, but as another form of healthcare. Sometimes it's practical, like a ride home or someone taking notes. Sometimes it's emotional, like a steady presence when you don't want to go through it by yourself. However it looks, asking for support isn't weakness. It's strategy. It lightens the weight you've been asked to hold, and it reminds you that you're not in this on your own.

### *Let Yourself Lean on Someone*

Taking care of yourself doesn't mean doing it all by yourself. Sometimes the strongest move you can make is allowing someone else to step in, not to fix it, but to be with you. Support can look like a friend sitting on the phone with you while you wait for test results. A partner driving you home after a procedure. A parent dropping off soup. A group text cheering you on before you walk through the clinic door.

Think about what would actually feel good for you. Do you want someone to bring you food? To remind you of the questions you wanted to ask? To take notes during the visit? To check in the next day? Everyone's version of support is different, and you're allowed to ask for what you need.

You can even set the terms: "I don't need advice, I just need you to listen." Or, "Can you be the one to remember the instructions in case I forget?" This is advocacy too, within your own relationships.

Letting yourself lean on support doesn't make you less independent or less strong. It reminds you that you don't have to do this alone. And sometimes, that reminder is the care you need most.

### Prompts to Open the Conversation

Accepting support is one step. Inviting it out loud is another. Many of us were never taught how to talk openly about periods, pain, fertility, or menopause, even with the people closest to us. But silence doesn't serve you here. These conversation starters are a way to open the door.

Naming these experiences, sometimes for the first time, is what shifts the weight. The more you speak them aloud, the easier it becomes to share the load. If you're not sure where to begin, you can try starting with these suggestions:

- "I've realized I haven't shared much about this part of my health, and I'd like to start."
- "I'd like to tell you more about how ____ has been affecting me."
- "I've noticed ____ happening with my body, and I want you to understand what that feels like."
- "This experience has been heavier than I expected, and I need you to know how it's still with me."
- "I don't need you to fix anything. I just need you to listen and be here with me."

These aren't scripts you have to memorize. They're springboards. Pick one, adapt it, or let it spark your own words. What matters is breaking the silence. Because these aren't small conversations. They're the ones that turn reproductive healthcare from something you carry alone into something your relationship can hold with you. And those conversations ripple outward, strengthening the partnership itself.

### Your Body, Your Relationships

Reproductive healthcare doesn't just live in your body, it extends into your relationships. The cycle pain that interrupts your plans. Mood shifts that sneak in with hormonal changes. Fertility struggles that bring hope one day and heartbreak the next. Hot flashes that break up your sleep. Dryness or discomfort that makes intimacy more complicated.

Even the in-between moments—the waiting, the wondering, the not-knowing—can reshape how you connect. Each of these moments doesn't just test your body; they can test the balance of your partnership. They shape intimacy, communication, and the ways you and your partner move through both the big milestones and the small daily rhythms of life together.

You don't have to carry that alone. Naming what you're going through out loud is the first step toward connection. Talk about the cramps that sideline you. The hot flashes that interrupt your sleep. The way a pregnancy loss can feel like an earthquake in your body and your heart. When you put words to it, you invite your partner into the conversation instead of leaving them standing outside the door.

Then, be clear about what support looks like for you. Maybe it's having them track medication times so you don't have to. Maybe it's asking them to take the night shift with the baby so you can recover. Maybe it's saying, "I don't need solutions. I need you to sit with me while I cry." Support isn't about fixing. It's about showing up the way you ask.

And if you're in a partnership with a man, I've tried to take some of the mental load off you. There's a bonus chapter written just for him. A crash course in showing up for reproductive healthcare. Not as a fixer, but as a partner who listens, learns, and leans in. Will it make him an expert? No. But it will give him a foundation, a vocabulary, and a way to start carrying part of the load. So hand it over. Let him do some of the homework.

### *Reclaiming Your Body*

Medical care has a way of pulling you out of yourself. You hand over pieces of your story, your privacy, even your comfort, and sometimes you leave feeling like you don't fully belong to your own body anymore. That disconnection can be subtle, an offhand comment that lingers, or it can be sharp, like when a procedure leaves you shaken or unheard. Reclaiming your body is about gathering those pieces back. It's the work of reminding yourself that your body is yours first, not the system's.

### Mindful Moments

Every appointment asks something of you: your time, your story, your body. Even routine visits can leave you feeling a little out of sync, like you've been spoken about more than spoken to, or like pieces of yourself were handed over and not yet returned. Reclaiming your body is about gently bringing yourself back to center after those moments.

One way to do that is through mindfulness. At its core, mindfulness is simply the practice of paying attention to the present moment, without judgment, without rushing to the next thing. It can help before a visit, by grounding you so you walk in with a steadier sense of self. It can help during a visit, by giving you tools to notice your own reactions and slow down enough to ask for what you need. And it can help afterward, by easing the stress or disconnection that lingers once you leave the exam room.

**Try this:** Wherever you are—sitting, standing, or lying down—bring your attention to how your body is being supported. Notice the surface beneath you, the points of contact that remind you: you are held. Take a slow breath in, noticing the air as it enters. Exhale just as slowly, allowing your body to soften a little with the release. Then silently remind yourself, *I am here. This is my body. I am safe to take up space.*

This can be done whenever you feel yourself start to spiral. When you're sad, angry, or frustrated. At home, in bed, in the car, or in the clinic while waiting for your doctor to walk in the room. Even a few breaths like this can help bring you back into yourself.

### *Rest Is Radical*

The system is designed to wear you down. Short visits. Long waits. Endless insurance calls. The weight of not being believed. It's no accident that you feel exhausted. It takes energy just to keep showing up. Which is why rest isn't indulgence. It's resistance.

Rest says, I am not just a patient to be processed. I am a person with limits, and those limits matter. Rest says, I refuse to let a broken system take more from me than it already has.

Sometimes that rest looks like literal recovery: napping after a procedure, taking a day before diving back into work, letting your body be tired instead of pushing through. Sometimes it's emotional rest: stepping away from the research rabbit holes, putting the phone down, letting yourself not have all the answers for a little while.

And sometimes it's relational rest: pausing before booking the next appointment, giving yourself space to regroup before going back in.

Rest doesn't mean you're giving up. It means you're making sure you have enough of yourself left to return. It means you get to decide the pace, the timing, the terms.

In a world that expects you to keep pushing, resting is a radical act of self-preservation. It's a reminder that your body isn't just something to fix. It's something to care for. And you deserve that care as much as any treatment or procedure.

## Owning Your Story, Protecting Your Safety

The healthcare system keeps records, but those records aren't always written with you in mind. Providers chart from their perspective. Insurance companies track only what they'll cover. And sometimes, the system doesn't just overlook your story, it turns against you, treating your health as suspicion instead of care. That's why it matters to keep your own account and to know your rights. One gives you clarity and leverage; the other gives you protection.

*Your Care File*

One of the most powerful tools you can carry is your own record of care. Providers write from their perspective. Insurance companies log what they'll cover. What's missing is your version of the story.

That's where your care file comes in. It doesn't have to be complicated. It can be a notebook, a notes app, or a folder on your computer. What matters is that it's yours. Write down what happened at each visit: what was said, what was done, how it felt. Save copies of test results, procedure notes, after-visit summaries, and bills. Screenshots suffice. If something doesn't line up, or if you ever need to push back, you'll have your own record to lean on. Think of it like keeping the receipts. You have your own paper trail.

Here's the hard truth: most clinics and hospitals run on different electronic record systems that don't talk to each other. Your new doctor may not see the labs you just had done. A specialist may not know what your primary care provider recommended. It's fragmented, and frustrating. Which is why keeping your own file matters even more. You get to be the captain of your care and the connector of the dots.

## Protecting Yourself in Unsafe Systems

Most of the time, medical visits are about getting care, not bracing for suspicion. But in today's landscape, there are moments when the system doesn't just fail you. It turns against you. Between 2000 and 2020, at least 61 documented cases in 26 states involved people investigated or arrested for their pregnancy outcomes, including miscarriages and self-managed abortions. And this was *before* the fall of *Roe v. Wade*. Many were charged not under abortion laws, but under statutes like child abuse or homicide. Laws never meant to police pregnancy.

This should never happen. But since we live in a country where police and prosecutors misuse their power and the law, it is critical to know how to keep yourself and your loved ones safe. That reality doesn't mean you shouldn't seek care, it means you deserve to know how to protect yourself while doing it.

If your care ever starts to feel unsafe, if questions shift from supportive to suspicious, remember this: you still have rights. You do not owe anyone every detail of what happened to you. You do not have to hand over your phone, your search history, or your private conversations. And if law enforcement or hospital staff ask questions that feel more like an interrogation than care, you do not have to answer. You have the right to remain silent. You have the right to a lawyer. And if someone tells you that silence equals guilt, they are wrong. And it means you may be at legal risk.

If this feels hard to believe, it isn't just theory. It's happening now. I spoke with Kylee Sunderlin, the legal services director who oversees If/When/How's Repro Legal Helpline. She told me, "Abortion, pregnancy loss, and birth are all parts of people's reproductive lives. And no one should fear criminalization for going to their healthcare provider. People deserve compassion and care, not suspicion and punishment."

Kylee's words stay with me because they're both a warning and a call to action. She has sat with the people living this reality, and she's also reminding us that no one should have to.

Protecting yourself isn't secrecy. It's survival. It's the recognition that the system doesn't always meet pregnancy with compassion, and that you deserve safety as much as you deserve care.

Knowing your rights isn't about living in fear. It's about standing steady in a world that sometimes wavers around you. Because your health is not a crime. And your body is not evidence.

## Carrying This Forward

Taking care of yourself isn't separate from healthcare. It *is* healthcare. Every time you ask for support, invite your partner into the conversation, take a moment to reclaim your body, rest instead of push, or write down your own version of what happened, you're building something powerful. You're building a kind of care that no clinic or insurance company can take away from you. None of this erases the brokenness of the system. But it does mean you walk into it differently: steadier, clearer, harder to dismiss. That's what this book is about. Not giving you a perfect path through healthcare, but giving you tools to make sure your needs don't get lost inside it.

Because your body is not just a site of treatment. It's the center of your life. And caring for it, on your terms, is part of what you deserve.

# Chapter 17

# Lessons from Abroad

*How Global Models Reveal What's Possible, and How to Bring Those Lessons Home*

Sometimes the clearest way to see what's wrong at home is to step outside of it. The United States spends more on healthcare than any other nation in the world, but our results tell a very different story. Our maternal mortality rate is among the worst of all wealthy countries.

So why should you care what happens abroad? Because it reveals what's possible. It shows us that better outcomes aren't some unattainable dream, they're happening right now, in real healthcare systems serving millions of people.

When you realize how much of what feels "normal" in the United States is actually not, it cracks something open. A rushed visit that ends before your questions do isn't the global standard. In other countries, new parents are supported by daily postpartum home visits, not left to navigate recovery alone. Paid leave is treated as essential to healing and bonding, not as a privilege to be negotiated with your employer. Pelvic floor therapy is offered automatically, not only if you beg insurance to cover it. And menopause, something every woman will face if she lives long enough, is built into routine care instead of treated like an afterthought. These aren't universal truths. They're uniquely American choices.

And once you see that, you can start asking different questions. You can look at your own care and say, "Why not here? Why not me?" Why can't I have continuity with the same provider? Why can't postpartum recovery be treated as essential instead of optional? Why should access to basic reproductive health depend on my state, my income, or my insurance coverage?

This isn't about pretending that importing another country's system is realistic overnight. It's about recognizing patterns that consistently lead to better outcomes—continuity of care, midwifery integration, parental leave, cultural responsiveness—and carrying those lessons back into your own exam room. Knowing what's possible elsewhere arms you with both perspective and power.

Other countries aren't perfect. They have their own shortages, wait times, and inequities. But they also prove that structure matters. They show us that policies, training, and priorities shape whether patients feel dismissed or cared for, supported or abandoned. And they remind us that the system we live under is the result of choices. Choices we have to be aware of and choices we can push to change.

## The Cost of Care: Affordability and Access

Having a baby in the United States is not just physically demanding, it's also financially punishing. Even with insurance, patients often face copays, deductibles, out-of-network fees, and surprise bills that pile up fast. A 2020 Health Affairs study found that women with private insurance paid an average of $4,500 out-of-pocket for pregnancy, delivery, and postpartum care. For families with high-deductible plans, the bill was much higher. For the uninsured, costs are staggering: a "routine" vaginal birth averages more than $18,000, while a cesarean section averages $26,000.

The financial weight has real consequences. Patients delay prenatal care because they can't afford the first bill. They skip ultrasounds or recommended labs. Some forgo continuity altogether, seeing whichever provider their insurance covers that month. And some avoid seeking care entirely, hoping nothing goes wrong.

Contrast that with the United Kingdom. Through the National Health Service (NHS), every pregnancy-related visit, ultrasound, and test is free at the point of service. Patients don't weigh groceries against the next appointment. They don't postpone prenatal visits until they can scrape together enough cash. Research shows that when cost isn't in the way, people start prenatal care earlier and attend more consistently. And earlier care means safer care. Complications are caught sooner, risks are managed earlier, and outcomes improve.

In the Nordic countries of Finland, Sweden, Norway, and Denmark, universal health coverage ensures care is accessible without financial burden. But it doesn't stop there. Paid, job-protected parental leave means families aren't forced back to work before they've healed. Hospital and community systems provide lactation support, home visiting programs, and postpartum recovery services at no cost. The result: healthier parents, lower infant mortality, and stronger maternal recovery. Finland's maternal mortality rate is 3 per 100,000 live births, compared to 19 in the United States. That gap is not about Finnish mothers being healthier or Finnish doctors working harder, it's about structure.

## *What This Means for You*

You may not be able to snap your fingers and turn the US healthcare system into the NHS or the Nordic model, but you can use this knowledge to shape your own experience.

Affordability elsewhere proves that the high costs you face here aren't inevitable, they're choices our system has made. And that perspective can help you take back some control.

Start by knowing what your insurance actually covers. Ask directly about maternity benefits: are prenatal vitamins, breast pumps, or lactation visits included? What about postpartum physical therapy (PT) or mental health support? Many people only discover after the fact that these services were covered all along. But only if they had asked.

Then, press your employer about leave. Even if your workplace isn't required to offer paid parental leave, some companies provide it voluntarily. Ask human resources (HR) what policies exist. And if there's nothing formal in place, you may still be able to negotiate short-term disability coverage, flexible scheduling, or the use of accrued sick or vacation days to buy yourself more recovery time.

Beyond insurance and work benefits, look for community-based supports. In many states, programs modeled after Nordic-style postpartum services do exist: Women, Infants and Children breastfeeding consultants, state-funded home visiting programs, or local nonprofits that provide free doulas and postpartum care. Your hospital's social worker or your local health department can often point you toward resources you might not know to look for.

Don't assume financial barriers can't be challenged. If you receive a surprise bill, request an itemized statement and ask the hospital to review the charges. Patients in the United States have successfully appealed thousands of dollars in "routine" charges simply by questioning them.

And finally, plan for costs the same way you plan for birth itself. If you're budgeting for diapers and a crib, add a line for healthcare expenses. Call your insurance company early in pregnancy to ask what you'll be responsible for at delivery. Knowing ahead of time not only helps you avoid shocks but also prepares you to push back if something doesn't add up.

Affordability isn't just about numbers. It shapes when you get care, how consistently you receive it, and whether you can walk into an appointment without bracing for a bill you can't pay. Other countries prove that financial stress doesn't have to be part of pregnancy. Here, it often is. But by naming it, planning for it, and challenging it when you can, you put yourself back in the driver's seat.

## What Care Looks Like: Standards and Transparency

In the United States, prenatal care is a patchwork. What you get depends on your state, your hospital, your insurance, and sometimes even the individual provider you happen to see that day. One patient may be offered multiple ultrasounds; another, just one. One clinic may build mental health screening into every visit; another may never mention it. There's no single national standard that guarantees a consistent level of care. For patients, that means you can walk out of an appointment never knowing if you actually received the full scope of what's recommended, or if you just got the version your provider, clinic, or insurer happened to deliver.

Contrast that with the United Kingdom. The National Institute for Health and Care Excellence (NICE) publishes detailed, evidence-based guidelines that spell out exactly what care should include at each stage of pregnancy. Providers are expected to follow them, and patients can read them, too. If a patient isn't offered something that's standard in the guidelines, say, a blood pressure check at every visit or a screening for gestational diabetes, they can point directly to the NICE guidance and ask why. That transparency doesn't just improve consistency; it builds trust. Patients know the benchmarks, and they know when care falls short.

In the United States, no such national playbook exists. ACOG (the American College of Obstetricians and Gynecologists) publishes guidelines, but they're often treated as professional recommendations, not enforceable standards. And because patients rarely see them, there's little transparency about what you should expect. That lack of clarity leaves too much room for gaps and inequities.

*What This Means for You*

You may not have the guidelines spelled out in plain language, but you can still use the same principle, know what the standard should be, and hold your care to it. That starts with asking directly. Try "What's the standard of care for this stage of pregnancy?" or "What do national guidelines recommend for someone like me?" A good provider should be able to tell you not just what they're doing, but why.

You can also do some homework on your own. ACOG, the US Preventive Services Task Force, and the Centers for Disease Control all publish guidelines online. They're not exactly light reading, but even skimming the basics will give you a sense of what's typical. That way, if something isn't offered, you'll notice.

And if you do spot a gap, don't be afraid to bring it up. You can frame it in a way that shows you're informed without being confrontational. Simple questions can open the door to important conversations.

Finally, remember you can use documentation as leverage. If a provider refuses a recommended test or screening, ask them to note the reason in your chart. Having it written down often changes the dynamic, and it protects you if something is missed later.

Standards matter because they turn healthcare from a guessing game into something you can rely on. Other countries prove that when expectations are consistent and public, outcomes improve. Here, the guidelines exist, but they're harder to see. By learning what they are and asking directly, you can bring those standards into the room with you and make them work in your favor.

## Culturally Responsive Care

Healthcare isn't just about tests and treatments, it's about whether the system sees you, hears you, and respects who you are. When care is blind to culture, patients disengage. When it's rooted in identity and community, outcomes improve.

In New Zealand, maternity care is organized through a Lead Maternity Carer. Patients choose a midwife or general practitioner (GP) who coordinates all their care throughout pregnancy and the postpartum period. After birth, your midwife will continue visiting you and your baby at home for up to six weeks. Only then is care transferred to the Well Child service and your GP for ongoing follow-up. For Māori families, this model is strengthened by culturally rooted programs that center family, honor traditional practices, and train providers in cultural safety. These efforts have helped improve engagement and outcomes in communities that have long been underserved.

Canada is also working to repair harm by restoring Indigenous midwifery programs. After decades of colonial policies that stripped away traditional practices and forced birth away from Indigenous communities, new programs are rebuilding local, culturally anchored models of care. The goal isn't only medical safety, it's dignity, trust, and keeping care close to home.

These examples prove that when healthcare honors identity and culture, patients engage earlier, stay connected longer, and trust the system more. And the reverse is also true: when care ignores culture, mistrust grows, leading to later entry into care, higher complication rates, and worse outcomes.

### *What This Means for You*

In the United States, culturally responsive care often comes down to the individual provider, the clinic, or the hospital. Not the system as a whole. That's a hard truth, because it means your experience may vary dramatically depending on where you go. But it also means you can, and should, ask the questions that help you gauge whether a provider will see and respect you.

Start with something direct: "How do you make care inclusive for patients like me?" The answer matters. Do they talk about specific practices, like using trained interpreters, incorporating family members into visits if you want them there, or asking about cultural or religious practices that shape your care preferences? Do they mention training in implicit bias or trauma-informed care? Or do they gloss over the question with something vague like, "We treat everyone the same"?

That response is data. If a provider can't answer clearly, or worse, dismisses the question, it tells you something important about how safe or supported you may feel under their care. And that's not something you should ignore.

If the answer feels incomplete, consider looking elsewhere. Community health centers, tribal clinics, LGBTQ+ clinics, or practices that explicitly advertise culturally competent or affirming care are often better equipped to meet diverse needs. Don't be afraid to seek out providers who name inclusivity as part of their mission. That usually means they've thought about it, built systems on it, and are more likely to follow through.

Culturally responsive care isn't an optional extra. It can mean the difference between getting a diagnosis early or late, trusting a treatment plan or walking away from it, feeling respected or feeling invisible. When care honors your identity, you're more likely to engage fully, ask questions openly, and get the outcomes you deserve.

Because at the end of the day, this isn't about being "nice." It's about safety, dignity, and trust. And every patient deserves that without exception.

## Support After Birth—Postpartum and Parental Leave

In the United States, postpartum care is almost nonexistent. For most people, it's one visit at six weeks, if it's even covered by insurance. That single check is supposed to clear you to resume sex, exercise, and sometimes even work, as if the massive physical, emotional, and hormonal shifts of birth could be neatly tied up in six weeks. And because the United States has no guaranteed paid parental leave, most parents are back at work within weeks. Still bleeding, still healing, still learning how to feed their baby. Forced to pretend they're fine.

I know this firsthand. I worked in an OB-GYN office while birthing my own babies. I had three separate maternity leaves. And every one of them was unpaid. I cared for patients all day, watching them navigate the same system I was living in, and then went home to figure out how to recover, mother, and pay the bills at the same time. It felt like the system asked me to split myself in two: a clinician who knew better and a mother just trying to survive.

In the United States, what you get after birth depends on your zip code, your insurance, and your employer. Some states have invested in home visiting programs or Medicaid extensions that cover a full year postpartum. Others still cut patients off at six weeks, or less. Some states guarantee a few weeks of paid family leave; others offer none at all. It's a patchwork of policies that determines whether you have a safety net or nothing. And that patchwork is unfair. Your access to recovery and bonding time shouldn't depend on which side of a state border you live on.

Other countries prove this isn't the only way. In the Nordic nations parents receive paid, job-protected leave for months, not weeks. Hospital systems are structured to support breastfeeding from the start: skin-to-skin contact is standard, lactation consultants are universally available, and community programs continue after discharge. Not surprisingly, over 90% of parents initiate breastfeeding, and many continue for months.

France takes another approach that should be universal: pelvic floor rehabilitation. Postpartum patients are routinely prescribed 10 to 20 sessions of physical therapy, fully covered by national health insurance. The goal is prevention, not crisis management, addressing incontinence, prolapse, and pain before they become lifelong problems. In the United States, pelvic floor therapy is often out of pocket, requires a referral, and isn't even mentioned unless you know enough to ask for it.

## *What This Means for You*

Don't wait for a 2 a.m. meltdown to get help. Ask for lactation support early. Whether you're nursing, bottle-feeding, or doing both, you deserve hands-on guidance. Often lactation consultants are not offered unless you ask.

Look into whether your state offers home visiting programs or whether local nonprofits provide free doulas or postpartum care. In some states, Medicaid covers a year of postpartum visits and support. In others, coverage ends after six weeks. This inconsistency is one of the deepest failures of our system. But it also means that resources may exist where you are, even if they're not widely advertised. Ask your provider, your hospital's social worker, or your local health department what's available.

Don't accept "you're fine" at six weeks. Healing takes longer. Ask for pelvic floor/postpartum physical therapy early, even if nothing feels "wrong." Sure, urinary leakage is common, but peeing your pants every time you sneeze is no way of life.

If your workplace doesn't provide formal parental leave, press HR about alternatives. Some companies quietly offer short-term disability coverage, flexible scheduling, or the option to use sick and vacation days to extend recovery time. Even a few extra weeks can make a huge difference when you're healing from childbirth, adjusting to a newborn, and figuring out your new normal.

And when it comes to costs, remember that you can push back. If you're billed for services you thought were covered, request an itemized bill and question the charges. Patients in the United States have successfully appealed thousands of dollars in "routine" costs simply by refusing to take them at face value.

Postpartum recovery shouldn't be a white-knuckle sport or a benefit that depends on your state line. It should be recognized, and supported, as the critical time period that it is. Other countries treat recovery as essential: funded, staffed, built into routine care. Here, it's fragmented, inconsistent, and too often missing. Name what you need, plan early, and push where you can. PT, lactation support, home visits, time off. Every ask moves you closer to the care and time you deserve. Every pushback chips away at the broken logic that parents in the United States should just "make do."

## Sex Education and Contraception Abroad

Reproductive health doesn't start in the delivery room. It starts long before, with the information (or misinformation) people are given about their own bodies. And here, the United States shows some of its deepest cracks.

In the Netherlands, sex education begins in pre-kindergarten, is consistent nationwide, and covers more than just anatomy. Kids learn about relationships, consent, communication, and pleasure in an age-appropriate way. The results are striking: Dutch teens start having sex later than US teens, use contraception more reliably when they do, and have far lower rates of unintended pregnancy and sexually transmitted infections.

Sweden has a similar approach: mandatory, comprehensive sex education in schools that is medically accurate and LGBTQ+ inclusive. Students are taught not only the "mechanics" of sex but also how to build respectful, healthy relationships.

Contrast that with the United States, where there are no national standards at all. What you get depends entirely on your state, or even your school district. I sit on the sex ed advisory board for my own school district in Michigan, and I recently learned they actually require clergy members to hold seats on the board. Think about that: decisions about what kids learn about their bodies are being shaped not just by educators or health professionals, but by clergy.

Some states do require comprehensive, evidence-based sex ed. Others go the opposite way, mandating "abstinence-only" or "abstinence-plus" programs that push waiting until marriage while downplaying, or outright misrepresenting, contraception. In 29 states, abstinence is legally required to be "stressed" in sex ed, and in many places, it's the only message students hear.

The result is predictable: huge gaps in knowledge. And those gaps show up in outcomes: higher teen pregnancy rates, higher sexually transmitted infection rates, and lower contraceptive use compared to countries where sex ed is consistent, evidence-based, and honest.

Contraceptive access follows a similar pattern. In France and the United Kingdom, contraception is treated as a core part of healthcare. In France, birth control pills and emergency contraception are free to anyone under 26. In the United Kingdom, all contraception, including intrauterine devices, implants, and emergency contraception, is free through the National Health Service. The focus isn't on moralizing; it's on preventing unintended pregnancies and giving people agency over their reproductive lives.

The United States, by contrast, has turned contraception into a political battleground. While the Affordable Care Act requires most insurance plans to cover contraception without out-of-pocket costs, loopholes and legal challenges remain. Access still depends heavily on your insurance, your income, and your state. For example, in some states pharmacists can prescribe birth control pills directly; in others, you still need to see a physician, adding time, cost, and barriers.

### *What This Means for You*

If your school pushed abstinence-only, skipped over contraception, or left out conversations about consent and pleasure, you're not alone. Millions of people in the United States were handed half-truths or no information at all. And for many, it wasn't just schools. You may have grown up in a religious or conservative household where sex was shamed, where curiosity was treated as sin, and where silence or fear took the place of honest conversations. That kind of stigma doesn't just disappear when you become an adult. It sticks, and it takes active, intentional deprogramming to undo.

But none of that means you're stuck with the gaps or the shame. You can take it on yourself to do the learning now that you never got. There are excellent resources online that walk through everything from contraception to healthy relationships to pleasure-based sex education. It's never too late to learn those lessons. And, in fact, learning them now can be deeply freeing. It gives you the confidence to advocate for yourself in healthcare, to have clearer conversations in your relationships, and to reclaim the parts of your body and sexuality that were once dismissed or stigmatized.

Seek out sex-positive clinicians. And when it comes to contraception, asking sharp questions makes a difference. Try: "Is this method fully covered under my plan? If not, what are my covered options?" Sometimes coverage exists but won't be offered unless you press. And because access depends on your state, it's worth asking: "Does my state allow pharmacists to prescribe birth control?" Knowing the answer could save you time, cost, and barriers.

The bottom line: sex education and contraception aren't luxuries. They're the foundation of reproductive health. If you didn't get what you needed as a teenager, you can still claim it now. Learn, ask, push. Those steps aren't just about filling the gaps, they're about refusing to let the system decide what you get to know about your own body.

## Carrying the Lessons Home

Looking beyond our borders isn't about wishing you lived somewhere else. It's about refusing to accept that what you're handed here is the best you can hope for. Other countries show us that the shape of care—the length of a visit, the cost of a test, the support you get after birth—isn't random. It's designed. Which means it can be redesigned.

That knowledge changes how you move through the system. It gives you permission to say, "This isn't inevitable. This isn't good enough. I deserve better." It helps you recognize when you're being shortchanged, and it arms you with sharper questions to ask in the exam room, in HR meetings, and at the ballot box.

You can't change US healthcare overnight. But you can change the way you show up in it: more informed, less willing to settle, and more connected to the reality that things can be different. And every time you push back, even a little, you're not just advocating for yourself. You're reminding the system, and the people around you, that "normal" is not the same as "enough."

# Chapter 18

# This Isn't Extra; This Is Your Right

*How to Take Everything You've Learned and Use It to Get the Care You Deserve*

By now you've seen the pattern: training gaps that erase whole chapters of care, insurance models that dictate treatment more than medicine does, and cultural biases that decide whose pain gets believed. You know the harm isn't accidental, it's designed into the system.

So let's say this clearly, one last time: the failures you've faced were not about your strength, your worth, or your ability to "advocate better." They were about a system that was not built with you in mind. A system that still rewards speed over listening, compliance over curiosity, billing codes over dignity.

If you've walked out of an appointment asking yourself, *Did I not push hard enough? Should I have said it differently?*, that is the conditioning talking. It's the internalized training of a culture that convinces patients—especially women, queer people, Black and Brown individuals—that when care falls short, it must be their fault. That story doesn't come out of nowhere; it's built on society's broader failure to empower women, to treat their pain as real, their choices as valid, and their voices as authoritative in their own healthcare.

But my hope is that you see it differently now. That you recognize how what once felt like a personal shortcoming is actually the result of a system built this way on purpose. Your struggles aren't isolated. You are not alone.

Now you have the concepts and some of the tools. This isn't about basics anymore. It's about applying them. It's about naming the truth without apology. Refusing to carry shame that was never yours. And turning that clarity into leverage. Because when you stop blaming yourself, you free up the energy to direct blame where it belongs. And you learn how to use your voice strategically, not self-consciously.

You were never the problem. You are the pressure point. You are the disruption. And you are the reminder that a system that works against its own patients is failing.

## You Deserve More Than the Bare Minimum

Respect. Time. Pain relief. Clear answers. Affirming care. These aren't luxuries, they're the baseline. Expecting them doesn't make you "difficult" or "high maintenance." It makes you human. Every time someone dismisses your pain or minimizes your questions, it's a reflection of their training, not your value. You deserve care that treats you like a whole person. Not a chart. Not a billing code.

And here's the deeper truth: when you accept less than that baseline, the system counts on it. Healthcare has been built on the quiet compliance of patients who are told that endurance is noble and questioning is disruptive. But bare minimum care isn't neutral. It's harmful. It creates delays in diagnosis, worsens outcomes, and drives people away from care altogether.

So let's stop calling this "good enough." A rushed 10-minute visit isn't good enough. An intrauterine device insertion without pain relief isn't good enough. Being told "it's just stress" when your symptoms point to something more isn't good enough. Dignity, time, and clear answers are not extras to be granted when convenient, they are the very definition of competent care.

And when you demand that baseline, you're not only protecting yourself, you're raising the bar for everyone who comes after you. Your insistence becomes its own form of quality control, a quiet but powerful check on a system that was never built to get it right in the first place. Each time you hold that line, you push healthcare to measure itself against what it was always supposed to honor: the humanity of the people it serves.

You deserve more. It is a fundamental truth, a standard. And the minute you internalize that truth, you stop negotiating against yourself, and you start negotiating against the system. Once you accept that, the next step is carrying that truth and your trust in yourself with you into the rooms where decisions about your body are actually made.

## Claiming Space Inside the Clinic Walls

The system may feel abstract until you're in a paper gown. That's the moment when everything you've learned here—the questions, the scripts, the mindset shifts—comes into play. Self-advocacy isn't just theory. It's practice, in real time, with your own body on the line.

Inside the clinic, you have every right to slow the pace, to ask for clarity, to request comfort measures, and to refuse what doesn't sit right. That's not being "difficult." That's exercising ownership over your own health. The culture of medicine has long trained patients, especially women, to be polite, grateful, compliant. But gratitude doesn't get you better care. Clarity does. Boundaries do. A well-timed question does.

Claiming space doesn't have to mean confrontation. Sometimes it's as simple as asking, "Can you repeat that in plain language?" or "What other options do I have?" Sometimes it's pausing a procedure until you feel ready, or reminding the provider, "I'd like for you to explain each step as we go." Sometimes it's choosing to walk away and seek a second opinion. Each of these is a form of reclaiming power in a space that has historically denied it.

And remember: you don't have to do this flawlessly. You don't have to get every word right. What matters is that you show up prepared to be more than passive. Every time you assert yourself, even in small ways, you bend the culture of medicine away from silence and toward accountability.

Inside those walls, your body is not just a case. It's not just a chart. It's you. And you are allowed to be more than compliant. You are allowed to be heard.

## Silence Keeps Us Isolated; Conversation Creates Power

You don't have to do this alone. In fact, you shouldn't do this alone. Self-advocacy matters, but collective advocacy is where power multiplies.

Start conversations. Not just about the easy parts of healthcare but also about the parts that hurt, confuse, or enrage you. Tell a friend what happened when your pain was dismissed. Ask another parent at the bus stop if their teen's doctor ever mentioned consent or contraception. Share the script that finally helped you get through an appointment without being silenced. Bring these stories into the open: on soccer sidelines, in group chats, across kitchen tables.

Because silence is one of the system's greatest weapons. Silence isolates us. It convinces each of us that we're the only one struggling, the only one doubting, the only one afraid. Silence turns systemic failure into private shame. But the moment we say it out loud, the illusion cracks. We see how many of us are carrying the same story.

And that's where power lives. Not in perfection, not in enduring pain quietly, but in naming the patterns together. What once felt like a personal flaw suddenly reveals itself as a collective wound.

What was once whispered becomes common knowledge. What felt personal becomes political. What felt shameful becomes solidarity.

Advocacy is exhausting if you do it alone. That's why community matters. When you tell your story, you light the way for someone else. When you hear theirs, you realize you're not crazy, not weak, and not alone. Conversation doesn't just connect us, it builds pressure. Every story swapped makes it harder for the system to claim "this is rare." Every script shared makes it harder for the next provider to brush off the next patient. Every parent who admits, "I wasn't offered pain relief" makes it harder for the next generation to accept that as normal.

Silence protects the system. Conversation disrupts it. And community sustains it. Together, we don't just survive the failures of healthcare, we create the leverage to change it.

## Breaking the Silence, Building the Future

The impact doesn't stop with us. Every time we speak openly about our bodies, our care, and our rights, we model something different for the next generation. When kids and teens see parents and adults talking honestly about reproductive health—not whispering, not hiding, not treating it as taboo—they grow up knowing these conversations belong at the dinner table, not just behind closed doors in a clinic.

If you're a parent, your opportunities extend into your child's care as well. You can model these same behaviors in their health appointments: asking questions, making space for their voice, and treating their concerns as valid. When your child sees you advocate, they learn it's not just allowed, it's expected. When they watch you ask for clarity or request real pain relief, they understand that their comfort and dignity matter in every exam room they'll enter for the rest of their lives.

Breaking the silence now means our children won't have to unlearn the same shame. They'll inherit a different baseline. One where questions are welcomed, care is expected, and dignity isn't up for debate.

And that's how culture shifts. Not just for us, but for everyone who comes after us. The legacy we leave isn't only in the policies we fight for or the lawsuits that change the law. It's in the everyday conversations that strip away shame and replace it with solidarity. It's in the expectation we hand down to the next generation: that care must be honest, competent, and affirming, that it must finally meet people as they are and as they deserve to be treated.

## Reproductive Rights Should Not Be Partisan

As I said at the start of this book, reproductive healthcare shouldn't be about left or right, red or blue. It's about dignity. It's about whether people can trust their bodies and their care. Every single person deserves safe, respectful, evidence-based healthcare. No matter their politics, their income, their religion, or their zip code.

The truth is, reproductive healthcare has been turned into a political football, but the reality on the ground is not abstract. It's a patient who can't get a miscarriage treated in the emergency room. It's a teenager who has to drive hours just to find birth control. It's a parent who can't afford a mammogram until their cancer is already advanced. None of those moments ask for your party affiliation. They ask whether you'll be met with compassion, skill, and timely care, or whether you'll be left to suffer because the system decided you weren't worth it.

Reproductive rights are not a "women's issue." They shouldn't be a partisan wedge. They are the baseline of health, safety, and equality. As you've seen through this book, it's all related. Abortion care is miscarriage care. They're impossible to untangle. If you care about maternal mortality, you care about reproductive rights. If you care about strong families, you care about reproductive rights. If you care about people being able to work, study, and live free from fear of medical catastrophe, you care about reproductive rights.

And here's the deeper truth: this fight belongs to all of us.

Patients can't fix it alone. Providers can't fix it alone. Parents, partners, policymakers, and communities all have a role. Whether you identify as conservative or progressive, religious or secular, urban or rural—you deserve good care. Your loved ones deserve good care. And so does the stranger you'll never meet.

The fight for reproductive healthcare isn't about sides. It's about survival. It's about fairness. It's about building a culture where no one is punished for needing care and no one is silenced for demanding it. That will take all of us. Working not as partisans, but as people who believe that dignity in healthcare is nonnegotiable.

## Beyond OB-GYN: Taking These Tools into All of Your Care

The strategies you've practiced here, asking clear questions, slowing the pace, naming your needs, don't stop at OB-GYN visits. They belong in every part of your healthcare. Primary care checkups, urgent care, specialist consultations, even dental or vision appointments all carry the same risks of rushing, minimizing, or missing you. They also give you the same opportunities to hold the line.

When your primary care provider brushes past your concerns, you can ask them to pause and explain. When a specialist uses language you don't understand, you can request plain speech. When you feel pressured into a test or treatment without a clear reason, you can slow the process and ask about alternatives. These tools are not niche. They are universal. They are a language of dignity that applies wherever your body is in someone else's hands.

Advocacy in one part of your care life strengthens the others. The more you practice it, the sharper your instincts become. You start to notice when care is falling short sooner. You trust yourself to push back without guilt. And you carry the reminder that your worth doesn't shrink or expand depending on which office you're sitting in. You deserve competent, compassionate care everywhere, not just in OB-GYN practices.

## Practicing Empowerment in Everyday Life

Self-advocacy doesn't just live in exam rooms. It's a muscle you build everywhere, and the stronger it gets in daily life, the easier it becomes to use when the stakes are high. Think about the moments when you swallow discomfort because it feels easier than speaking up: a meal that isn't what you ordered or that nail color you didn't actually want. Those aren't trivial. They're practice.

Each time you name what isn't working, you prove to yourself that your voice matters. Each time you set a boundary in a relationship, a workplace, or a store, you remind yourself that your comfort counts. Boundaries can sound like, "I'm not available to take on extra work right now" or "I'd rather not discuss that topic today." They can be as simple as, "Please don't touch me without asking first," or "I need you to lower your voice if we're going to keep talking about this." They don't have to be dramatic to be powerful. They just have to be clear.

And here's something important: requesting a correction or setting a boundary doesn't have to be rude. You can put your foot down and still be kind. Kindness and clarity can absolutely coexist. When you approach self-advocacy this way, you not only make it easier on yourself, you also model for others that strength and compassion belong together. And that women can embody both fully.

Start where it feels manageable. Ask for your coffee order to be fixed. Say no to a coworker when your plate is already full. Ask for more support from your partner. It might feel awkward at first, but so does self-advocacy in healthcare. The more you practice, the more fluent you become. And over time, you stop carrying the fear of being "too much" and start carrying the clarity that you are enough.

Enough to ask for what you need without apology.

Enough to take up space in rooms that once made you feel small.

Enough to expect care that honors your dignity instead of testing your endurance.

Enough to know that boundaries are not selfish, they are necessary.

Enough to walk into any clinic and expect to be treated like a whole person.

When you move through the world with that clarity, you stop negotiating against yourself. You no longer shrink to fit broken models of care or relationships. You stop explaining away harm that was never yours to absorb. You begin to see self-advocacy not as a burden but as a birthright.

That is what changes everything: the steady, everyday insistence that you are worthy of respect, worthy of care, and worthy of being heard. And the more you embody that truth, the more impossible it becomes for the system, or anyone in it, to convince you otherwise.

This is how advocacy becomes not just a tactic but a way of moving through the world. You get used to hearing your own voice in moments of resistance. You get used to claiming space. And when it matters most, when your body, your health, your future are on the line, you'll know that you can do more than endure. You can speak. You can demand. You can expect more.

## Claiming What We Deserve

You've carried the weight of broken training, rushed visits, silenced trauma, denied pain, and systemic bias. You've seen how those cracks show up in real lives. Perhaps it's impacted your life. Your care. Or maybe that of a loved one. You're seeing how it shows up in real time and you're naming it out loud, maybe for the first time.

And now you hold something powerful: clarity, language, tools, and a sharper radar for the games and gaps. You know how to show up for yourself, how to protect your own care, and how to start conversations that shift culture.

This is where it all comes together. Not as theory, not as survival, but as a demand. A declaration. A reminder that what you deserve isn't "extra." It's the baseline. And claiming it is how we change everything.

I hope this book reminded you of something you never should've had to learn.

**You deserve more.**

More time. More trust. More clarity. More care.

You deserve providers who listen. Who believe you. You deserve systems that work for you, not against you. You deserve to feel safe in your body, and in the rooms where decisions are made about it.

This isn't just about reproductive healthcare. It's about reclaiming your place in a system and a society that was never built for you. And refusing to be quiet about it.

Every time you ask a better question. Every time you push back on a denial. Every time you say, "That didn't feel right" or "I'm going to need more from you," you shift the culture. You create cracks in a system that counts on silence. You send a message.

And we're not just doing this for ourselves. We're doing it for our best friends. For our sisters. In solidarity with our gender-expansive, nonbinary, and trans siblings. In honor of our mothers. Perhaps in memory of our grandmothers. And in preparation for our daughters, and all who will come after them.

We are done blaming ourselves for systemic failure. We are done being rushed, dismissed, and gaslit.

We are done shrinking to fit broken care models.

We're not just surviving this system. We're changing it. From the inside out.

And that change? It starts with you. It starts with us.

**Because We Deserve More.**

# Want More?

# The Workbook

*A Companion for the Road Ahead*

This book was written to validate your experiences, give you the context you've been missing, and hand you tools to advocate inside a system that too often shuts you out.

But reading is only the beginning. Walking into the exam room, remembering the right questions, and speaking up in real time, that takes practice. That's where the *We Deserve More Workbook* comes in.

The workbook is your hands-on guide. It takes the strategies from these chapters and puts them into practice with the following content:

- **Pre-visit planning pages** to define what matters most before you walk in
- **Scripts and prompts** to lean on when the words are hard to find
- **Reflection spaces** to process what went well, what didn't, and what you want to try differently
- **Scenario-based exercises** to rehearse for real-world moments

Think of this hardcover book as the *why*. The workbook is the *how*. The part you can carry with you, write in, fold over, highlight, and return to whenever the system feels overwhelming.

You'll find **10 core skills and 27 guided scenarios.** Each skill a practical, compassionate road map through the real reproductive healthcare challenges people face every day. The workbook spans identity-based navigation, cycle symptoms, pain and hormonal concerns, birth control, sexual health, fertility and family building, abortion care, pregnancy loss, and the structural barriers that shape care, including insurance gaps, rural access, and state-level restrictions. Every scenario includes scripts, strategies, and reflection space so you can walk into care prepared, and walk out with more of what you need. And because no one should have to navigate care alone, every scenario also includes a dedicated callout box written for support people: partners, parents, friends, or chosen family. These boxes give your people concrete ways to stand by you: what to say, how to advocate, when to step in, and how to help you feel less alone in the room.

Together, this book and the workbook are two halves of the same promise. The book validates your experiences and gives you the knowledge you've been missing. The workbook transforms that knowledge into action, offering space to plan, scripts to lean on, and strategies you can return to when care feels overwhelming. Because you don't just deserve to know more. You deserve a way forward. And the workbook will help. It features the following information:

**Part I: Core Skills:** Foundational tools that make every visit smoother and help you navigate your care with clarity and confidence.

1. **Your Medical Snapshot**
   A simple template to organize your history, meds, symptoms, and priorities.
2. **Making the Right Appointment**
   How to choose the correct visit type and make sure you're booked for it.

3. **Preparing for Your Annual Exam**
   What to expect, what to ask, and how to get your concerns addressed.
4. **Planning for a Problem Visit**
   How to describe symptoms clearly and advocate for real answers.
5. **Tracking Symptoms**
   A straightforward system for timing, patterns, and impact.
6. **The Art of Good Questions**
   How to ask questions that lead to real explanations, not one-word responses.
7. **Bringing Someone With You (or Not)**
   How to choose, prep, or set boundaries with a support person.
8. **Outlining Your "What Ifs"**
   Planning ahead for the unexpected so you're never caught off guard.
9. **Reflecting After a Visit**
   Tools to process what happened and clarify your next steps.
10. **When Care Doesn't Go Right**
    Scripts to redirect in the moment and guidance on when, and how, to find a new clinician.

**Part II: Scenarios:** Real-world situations where reproductive healthcare often falls short. Each with scripts, strategies, and guidance so you can walk into care prepared and walk out with more of what you need.

## Foundations of Care and Identity-Based Navigation

- Bringing Your Teen In for Their First Visit
- Being Overweight in the Exam Room
- Trans and Nonbinary Gynecological Care
- Navigating OB-GYN Care as a Black Woman or Birthing Person
- Navigating Gynecological Care with a History of Trauma
- Mental Health Deserves a Plan

**Cycle Symptoms, Hormonal Shifts, and Pain Concerns**
- Birth Control That Works for You
- When Your Bleeding Doesn't Make Sense
- Irregular Periods, Polycystic Ovary Syndrome (PCOS), and Getting Real Answers
- Endometriosis, Adenomyosis, and the Pain They Don't See
- Ovarian Cysts—When Pain, Pressure, and Uncertainty Collide
- Menopause Misinformation, HRT, and Being Taken Seriously

**Sex, Fertility, and Family Building**
- Sexual Health Beyond "Just Use Lube"
- Family Expansion Conversations That Don't Assume
- Aging and Egg Freezing: What You Should Know
- It's Time to Try: Getting Pregnant on Purpose
- Starting Infertility Conversations
- Queer Sex Ed: The Class We All Deserved
- Same-Sex Family Planning

**Abortion Care and Pregnancy Loss**
- Navigating Abortion Care by Choice
- Termination for Medical Reasons (TFMR)
- Selective Reduction in a Multifetal Pregnancy
- Miscarriage Management in and out of the ER

**Barriers and Safety**
- When You Don't Have Insurance
- When You Live in a Rural Area
- Living in a State with an Abortion Ban
- Navigating Reproductive Coercion, Abuse, or Control

The workbook isn't homework, it's a lifeline. Each page is designed to meet you in the messiness of real appointments, real decisions, and real emotions. It's a place to practice, to prepare, and to process. And over time, it becomes more than a guide, it becomes your record of strength, a reminder that you are not powerless in a system that too often makes you feel that way.

You deserve care that sees you, respects you, and responds to you. Until the system delivers on that promise, this workbook is here to help you hold the line.

# Bonus Chapter

# A Call In for Men

*The Power of Your Support in Reproductive Healthcare*

If you're reading this book for yourself, you've done the hard part. You've named that something in the system feels broken, and you've sought out tools to change how you move through it. But you don't have to carry this alone.

This bonus chapter is different. It's written with someone else in mind. A man who loves you, who wants to show up but may not know how.

So share it. Hand him the link to this section. Say, "Here's how you can be there for me." Because your care deserves to be a shared effort, not a solo act.

And if you're the man holding this now, consider it an invitation. Not to fix, not to take over, but to lean in. To listen. To learn. To stand steady in the moments when the system falters.

Change doesn't just come from exam tables and waiting rooms. Sometimes, it begins with the choice to show up for someone you love.

This chapter won't apply to everyone, and that's okay. This one was written just for men.

The following QR code scans to this chapter online:

Or go to the link: http://nikkivinck.com/formen

# Bonus Chapter

# A Call In for Those Who Wear White Coats

This book was written for your patients. But this section is for you. The clinicians. The ones holding the charts, writing the orders, walking into exam rooms where patients are bracing for dismissal or silence.

You worked hard for the initials after your name. You may know and truly feel that the system is broken. And yet you're still here, trying to do right by your patients in spite of it. This section is for you. Not to lecture, but to invite. Not to assign blame, but to open a door. This isn't about calling you out. It's about calling you in.

I'm deeply honored that you took the time to read this. I hope it felt helpful and worthwhile. Maybe it put words to frustrations you have felt but could not quite name. Maybe it helped you feel seen and validated. My hope is that it did not feel accusatory or make you feel targeted. If you have spent any time with this book at all, you are clearly part of the solution, not the problem. And for that, I am so thankful. This bonus chapter was written just for you.

The following QR code scans to this chapter online:

Or go to the link: http://nikkivinck.com/forclinicians

# References

## Chapter 2

Allen, J. T., Laks, S., Zahler-Miller, C., Rungruang, B. J., Braun, K., Goldstein, S. R., & Schnatz, P. F. Needs assessment of menopause education in United States obstetrics and gynecology residency training programs. *Menopause, 30*(10), 1002–1005. https://doi.org/10.1097/GME.0000000000002234

Brodsky, P. L. (2008). Where have all the midwives gone? *The Journal of Perinatal Education, 17*(4), 48–51. https://doi.org/10.1624/105812408X324912

Byrne, J., Straub, H., DiGiovanni, L., Collins, C., & Reame, N. (2014). Evaluation of ethics education in obstetrics and gynecology residency programs. *American Journal of Obstetrics and Gynecology, 210*(2), 171.e1–171.e8.

Christophers, B., Marr, M. C., & Pendergrast, T. R. (2022). Medical school admission policies disadvantage low-income applicants. *The Permanente Journal, 26*(2), 172–176.

March of Dimes. (2023). *Nowhere to go: Maternity care deserts across the US.* Author.

Morgan, H. K., Winkel, A. F., Standiford, T., Weavind, L., & Andriole, D. A. (2016). Readiness of medical students for obstetrics and gynecology residency: A national survey. *Obstetrics & Gynecology, 127*(5), 861–869.

Mutter, M., Sheinfeld, L., & Raymond, M. (2019). Obstetrics and gynecology residency training: A national survey of residents and program directors. *Journal of Graduate Medical Education, 11*(3), 292–299. https://doi.org/10.4300/JGME-D-18-00809.1

National Academies of Sciences, Engineering, and Medicine. (2025). *A new vision for women's health research: Transformative change at the National Institutes of Health.* National Academies Press.

Nayak, A. (2024, February 29). The history that explains today's shortage of Black midwives. *Time – Made by History.* https://time.com/6731376/black-midwives-shortage-history/

Sepulveda, D., & Varaklis, K. (2012). Implementing a multifaceted quality-improvement curriculum in an obstetrics-gynecology resident continuity-clinic setting: A 4-year experience. *Journal of Graduate Medical Education, 4*(2), 237–241. https://doi.org/10.4300/JGME-D-11-00158.1

Shields, K. E., & Lyerly, A. D. (2013). Exclusion of pregnant women from industry-sponsored clinical trials. *Obstetrics & Gynecology, 122*(5), 1077–1081.

Topcu, G., Cetin, S., & Sahinoglu, S. (2023). A global study on the abortion views and knowledge of trainee obstetricians and gynecologists. *International Journal of Gynecology & Obstetrics, 163*(2), 448–456.

Urban, R. R., He, H., Hardesty, M. M., & Goff, B. A. (2018). Obstetrics and gynecology residency training and preparation for fellowship: A survey of subspecialty fellows. *Obstetrics & Gynecology, 132*(4), 935–942.

World Health Organization. (2023, March). Endometriosis. https://www.who.int/news-room/fact-sheets/detail/endometriosis

Zemtsov, D., & Fitzgerald, J. E. F. (2025). Gynecologic surgery deserves its own residency. *JAMA Surgery, 160*(11), 1173–1174.

# Chapter 3

Ajjarrapu, A., Story, W. T., & Haugsdal, M. (2021). Addressing obstetric health disparities among refugee populations: Training the next generation of culturally humble OB/GYN medical providers. *Teaching and Learning in Medicine, 33*(3), 326–333.

American College of Obstetricians and Gynecologists (ACOG). (2019, October 28). Why OB-GYNs are burning out. https://www.acog.org/news/news-articles/2019/10/why-ob-gyns-are-burning-out

Association of American Medical Colleges (AAMC). (2022). *Differences in birthing experiences of LGBTQ+ and straight people.* Author.

Clark, L. E., Allen, R. H., Goyal, V., Raker, C., & Gottlieb, A. S. (2013). Reproductive coercion and co-occurring intimate partner violence in obstetrics and gynecology patients. *American Journal of Obstetrics and Gynecology, 208*(1), 31.e1–31.e7.

DeAndrade, S., Pelletier, A., Grossman, S., Lewis-O'Connor, A., Dutton, C., Royce, C. S., & Bartz, D. (2024). Trauma-informed care training in U.S. and Canadian Ob/Gyn residencies. *Violence Against Women, 31*(5), 1201–1212.

Donndelinger, S. (2025, April 22). Why lesbians face a maternal healthcare crisis. Uncloseted Media. https://unclosetedmedia.com

Duggan, M. P., Kodali, A. T., Panton, Z. A., Smith, S. M., Riew, G. J., Donaghue, J. F., Leya, G. A., & Briggs, L. G. (2023). Survey of nutrition education among medical students. *Journal of Wellness, 4*(2), Article 11.

Frazer, Z., McConnell, K., & Jansson, L. M. (2019). Treatment for substance use disorders in pregnant women: Motivators and barriers. *Drug and Alcohol Dependence, 205*, 107652.

Garbarino, A. H., Kohn, J. R., Coverdale, J. H., & Kilpatrick, C. C. (2019). Current trends in psychiatric education among obstetrics and gynecology residency programs. *Academic Psychiatry, 43*, 294–299.

Grindler, N. M., Allsworth, J. E., Macones, G. A., Kannan, K., Roehl, K. A., & Cooper, A. R. (2018). Persistent organic pollutants and early menopause in U.S. women. *PLoS One, 10*(1), e0116057.

Hardeman, R. R., Murphy, K. A., Karbeah, J., & Kozhimannil, K. B. (2018). Naming institutionalized racism in the public health literature: A systematic literature review. *Public Health Reports, 133*(3), 240–249.

Harris Wallace, B., Ford, C. D., & Baker, T. A. (2024). Advancing the inclusion of Black women in studies of menopause. *The Journals of Gerontology: Series A, 79*(2), glad284. https://doi.org/10.1093/gerona/glad284

Hartmann, K. E., Fonnesbeck, C., Surawicz, T., Gunderson, E., Jerome, R., Halladay, J., Lardi, C., & Nian, H. (2017). Management of uterine fibroids. *Comparative Effectiveness Review, 195* (AHRQ Publication No. 17(18)-EHC028-EF).

Human Rights Campaign Foundation. (2022). Healthcare Equality Index 2022: Executive summary. https://hrc.org/hei

Ireland, L. D., & Allen, R. H. (2016). Pain management for gynecologic procedures in the office. *Obstetrical & Gynecological Survey, 71*(2), 89–98.

Jones, J. M. (2021, February 24). LGBT identification rises to 5.6% in latest U.S. estimate. Gallup. https://news.gallup.com/poll/329708/lgbt-identification-rises-latest-estimate.aspx

Jones, J. M. (2025, February 20). LGBTQ+ identification in U.S. rises to 9.3%. Gallup. https://news.gallup.com/poll/656708/lgbtq-identification-rises.aspx

Kaiser Family Foundation. (2025). Americans' challenges with health care costs. https://www.kff.org/health-costs/issue-brief/americans-challenges-with-health-care-costs/

Kingsberg, S. A., & Simon, J. A. (2018). Female sexual dysfunction: Current trends and future directions. *International Journal of Women's Health, 10*, 353–364.

Laumann, E. O., Paik, A., & Rosen, R. C. (1999). Sexual dysfunction in the United States: Prevalence and predictors. *JAMA, 281*(6), 537–544.

Lederer, L. J., & Wetzel, C. A. (2014). The health consequences of sex trafficking and their implications for identifying victims in healthcare facilities. *Annals of Health Law, 23*(1), 61–91.

Morris, J., Clark, C., Reed, L., Pace, D., Cao, X., & Khanna, P. (2021). Healthcare provider knowledge, attitudes, and preferences in management of genitourinary syndrome of menopause in the Mid-South. *Menopause, 28*(11), 1239–1246. https://doi.org/10.1097/GME.0000000000001847

Obedin-Maliver, J., Goldsmith, E. S., Stewart, L., et al. (2011). Lesbian, gay, bisexual, and transgender-related content in undergraduate medical education. *JAMA, 306*(9), 971–977.

O'Laughlin, D. J., Strelow, B., Fellows, N., Kelsey, E., Peters, S., Stevens, J., & Tweedy, J. (2021). Addressing anxiety and fear during the female pelvic examination. *Journal of Primary Care & Community Health, 12*, 2150132721992195.

Postpartum Support International. (2023). *Perinatal mental health disorders: Prevalence and impact.*

Sekeres, M. A. (2025, June 23). As an oncologist, here's what I wish people knew about endocrine disruptors: What to know about everyday exposures to BPA, PFAS and phthalates. *The Washington Post.*

Veterans Health Administration. (2020). *Trauma-informed care implementation and outcomes in women's health settings.* Department of Veterans Affairs.

World Economic Forum. (2024). *The economic impact of menopause: Understanding workplace productivity and healthcare costs.* Author.

# Chapter 4

Allen, J. O., Solway, E., Kirch, M., Singer, D., Kullgren, J. T., Moïse, V., . . . & Malani, P. N. (2022). Experiences of everyday ageism and the health of older US adults. *JAMA Network Open, 5*(6), e2217240.

Badreldin, N., Grobman, W. A., & Yee, L. M. (2019). Racial disparities in postpartum pain management. *Obstetrics & Gynecology, 134*(6), 1147–1153.

Bauer, G. R., Scheim, A. I., Pyne, J., Travers, R., & Hammond, R. (2015). Intervenable factors associated with suicide risk in transgender persons: A respondent driven sampling study in Ontario, Canada. *BMC Public Health, 15*, 525.

Berrian, A. M., Douglass, C. H., Boakye, K. A., & Thompson, L. A. (2024). Barriers to quality healthcare among transgender and gender nonconforming adults. *Health Services Research, 60*(1), e14362.

Centers for Disease Control and Prevention (CDC). (2024, May 14). *Pregnancy-related deaths: Data and statistics.* US Department of Health and Human Services.

Centers for Disease Control and Prevention (CDC). (2025, April 3). Healthcare cost data. Disability and Health Data System (DHDS). https://www.cdc.gov/dhds/healthcare-cost-data/index.html

Chang, E. S., Kannoth, S., Levy, S., Wang, S. Y., Lee, J. E., & Levy, B. R. (2020). Global reach of ageism on older persons' health: A systematic review. *PLoS One, 15*(1), e0220857.

Diamond, L. C., Wilson-Stronks, A., & Jacobs, E. A. (2010). Do hospitals measure up to the national culturally and linguistically appropriate services standards? *Medical Care, 48*(12), 1080–1087.

Iezzoni, L. I., Rao, S. R., Ressalam, J., Bolcic-Jankovic, D., Agaronnik, N. D., Donelan, K., Lagu, T., & Campbell, E. G. (2021). Physicians' perceptions of people with disability and their health care. *Health Affairs, 40*(2), 297–306. https://doi.org/10.1377/hlthaff.2020.01452

Kagan, S. H., & Melendez-Torres, G. J. (2015). Ageism in nursing. *Journal of Nursing Management, 23*(5), 644–650.

Kcomt, L. (2020). Healthcare avoidance due to anticipated discrimination among transgender people: A call to create trans-affirmative environments. *SSM - Population Health, 11*, 100608.

Lawrence, B. J., Kerr, D., Pollard, C. M., Theophilus, M., Alexander, E., Haywood, D., & O'Malley, C. (2021). Weight bias among health care professionals: A systematic review and meta-analysis. *Obesity, 29*(11), 1802–1812.

Medicaid and CHIP Payment and Access Commission (MACPAC). (2021). Physician acceptance of new Medicaid patients: Findings from the National Electronic Health Records Survey.

Nguyen, B. T., & Lucero, J. (2018). Distribution of obstetrician–gynecologists and obstetric care in the United States. *Obstetrics & Gynecology, 132*(6), 1070–1076.

Petersen, E. E., Davis, N. L., Goodman, D., Cox, S., Syverson, C., Seed, K., Shapiro-Mendoza, C., Callaghan, W. M., & Barfield, W. (2019). Racial/ethnic disparities in pregnancy-related deaths—United States, 2007–2016. *Morbidity and Mortality Weekly Report, 68*(35), 762–765.

Pew Research Center. (2017). Facts on U.S. immigrants. https://www.pewresearch.org/race-and-ethnicity/2019/06/03/facts-on-u-s-immigrants-2017-data/

Puhl, R. M., & Brownell, K. D. (2006). Confronting and coping with weight stigma: An investigation of overweight and obese adults. *Obesity, 14*(10), 1802–1815.

Puhl, R. M., Peterson, J. L., & Luedicke, J. (2013). Fighting obesity or obese persons? Public perceptions of obesity-related health messages. *International Journal of Obesity, 37*(6), 774–782.

Reisner, S. L., Poteat, T., Keatley, J., Cabral, M., Mothopeng, T., Dunham, E., Holland, C. E., Max, R., & Baral, S. D. (2016). Barriers to health care for transgender individuals. *Current Opinion in Endocrinology, Diabetes, and Obesity, 23*(2), 168–171.

Stillman, M. D., Frost, K. L., Smalley, C., Bertocci, G., & Williams, S. (2017). Health care utilization and barriers experienced by individuals with spinal cord injury. *PM&R, 9*(9), 832–840.

World Health Organization. (2023). World report on disability. https://www.who.int/publications/i/item/world-report-on-disability

# Chapter 5

American College of Obstetricians and Gynecologists (ACOG). (n.d.). Implementing perinatal mental health screening. https://www.acog.org/programs/perinatal-mental-health/implementing-perinatal-mental-health-screening.

American Medical Association. (2025, April 24). Fixing prior auth: Nearly 40 prior authorizations a week is way too many. https://www.ama-assn.org/practice-management/prior-authorization/fixing-prior-auth-nearly-40-prior-authorizations-week-way

Braddock, C. H., Edwards, K. A., Hasenberg, N. M., Laidley, T. L., & Levinson, W. (1999). Informed decision making in outpatient practice: Time to get back to basics. *JAMA, 282*(24), 2313–2320.

Easter, R., Friedrich-Karnik, A., & Kavanaugh, M. L. (2024). Any restrictions on reproductive health care harm reproductive autonomy: Evidence from four states. Guttmacher Institute. 10.1363/2024.300471

Forouzan, K., & Guarnieri, I. (2023, December 19). *State policy trends 2023: In the first full year since Roe fell, a tumultuous year for abortion and other reproductive health care.* Guttmacher Institute.

Hamel, L., Norton, M., Pollitz, K., Levitt, L., Claxton, G., & Brodie, M. (2016, January). The burden of medical debt: Results from the Kaiser Family Foundation/*New York Times* medical bills survey. Kaiser Family Foundation. https://www.kff.org/health-costs/report/the-burden-of-medical-debt-results-from-the-kaiser-family-foundationnew-york-times-medical-bills-survey/

Kaiser Family Foundation. (2022a, June). Health care debt in the U.S.: The broad consequences of medical and dental bills. https://www.kff.org/health-costs/report/kff-health-care-debt-survey/

Kaiser Family Foundation (KFF). (2022b, February 16). Medicaid coverage for women. https://www.kff.org/womens-health-policy/issue-brief/medicaid-coverage-for-women/

Kaiser Family Foundation (KFF). (2023). Women's health insurance coverage and access to care.

Kaiser Family Foundation (KFF). (2024). Coverage and use of contraception and abortion services in the United States: A review of policy and access.

LendingTree. (2022, June 20). 33% don't know if employer covers fertility benefits. https://www.lendingtree.com/personal/fertility-treatments-survey/

March of Dimes. (2022). *Maternity care deserts report*. Author.

Medscape. (2024, January 24). Physician burnout & depression report 2024. https://www.medscape.com/slideshow/2024-lifestyle-burnout-6018669

Merritt Hawkins. (2022). 2022 Survey of physician appointment wait times and Medicare and Medicaid acceptance rates. https://www.merritthawkins.com

National Women's Law Center. (2023, September 20). Your health insurance company is gaslighting you—and breaking the law. https://nwlc.org/your-health-insurance-company-is-gaslighting-you-and-breaking-the-law/

# Chapter 6

American College of Obstetricians and Gynecologists (ACOG). (2021, June). Access to postpartum sterilization. https://www.acog.org/clinical/clinical-guidance/committee-opinion/articles/2021/06/access-to-postpartum-sterilization

Association of American Medical Colleges (AAMC). (2023). *Applications to OB/GYN residencies drop in states with abortion bans*. Author.

Cutler, A. S., Hale, C. M., Bennett, E., et al. (2025). Experiences of obstetrician-gynecologists providing pregnancy care after Dobbs. *JAMA Network Open, 8*(3), e252498. https://doi.org/10.1001/jamanetworkopen.2025.2498

Gill, J. M., Page, G. G., Sharps, P., & Campbell, J. C. (2008). Experiences of traumatic events and associations with PTSD and depression development in urban health care-seeking women. *Journal of Urban Health, 85*(5), 693–706.

Hasselbacher, L. A., Hebert, L. E., Liu, Y., & Stulberg, D. B. (2020). "My hands are tied": Abortion restrictions and providers' experiences in religious and non-religious health care systems. *Perspectives on Sexual and Reproductive Health, 52*(2), 107–115. https://doi.org/10.1363/psrh.12148

Menegay, M. C., Andridge, R., Rivlin, K., & Gallo, M. F. (2022). Delivery at Catholic hospitals and postpartum contraception use, five US states, 2015–2018. *Perspectives on Sexual and Reproductive Health, 54*(1) 5–11. https://doi.org/10.1363/psrh.12186

Phillips, K. A., Ospina, N. S., & Montori, V. M. (2019). Physicians interrupting patients. *Journal of General Internal Medicine, 34*(10), 1965. https://doi.org/10.1007/s11606-019-05247-5

Sabbath, E. L., McKetchnie, S. M., Arora, K. S., & Buchbinder, M. (2024). US obstetrician-gynecologists' perceived impacts of post-*Dobbs v. Jackson* state abortion bans. *JAMA Network Open, 7*(1), e2352109.

Shanafelt, T. D., West, C. P., Dyrbye, L. N., Sinsky, C., Trockel, M., Tutty, M., Carlasare, L. E., & Satele, D. V. (2022). Changes in burnout and satisfaction with work-life integration in physicians and the general U.S. working population between 2011 and 2021. *JAMA Health Forum, 3*(10), e224046.

Stulberg, D. B., Dude, A. M., Dahlquist, I., & Curlin, F. A. (2012). Obstetrician-gynecologists, religious institutions, and conflicts regarding patient-care policies. *American Journal of Obstetrics and Gynecology, 207*(1), 73.e1-5. https://doi.org/10.1016/j.ajog.2012.04.023

# Chapter 7

Ayers, S., Horsch, A., Garthus-Niegel, S., et al., & COST Action CA18211. (2024). Traumatic birth and childbirth-related post-traumatic stress disorder: International expert consensus recommendations for practice, policy, and research. *Women and Birth, 37*(2), 362–367.

Black, M. C., Basile, K. C., Breiding, M. J., Smith, S. G., Walters, M. L., Merrick, M. T., Chen, J., & Stevens, M. R. (2011). *The National Intimate Partner and Sexual Violence Survey (NISVS): 2010 Summary Report.* National Center for Injury Prevention and Control, Centers for Disease Control and Prevention.

Gorfinkel, L., Perlow, E., & Macdonald, S. (2021). The trauma-informed genital and gynecologic examination. *Canadian Medical Association Journal, 193*(28), E1090.

Irish, L., Kobayashi, I., & Delahanty, D. L. (2009). Long-term physical health consequences of childhood sexual abuse: A meta-analytic review. *Journal of Pediatric Psychology, 35*(5), 450–461. https://doi.org/10.1093/jpepsy/jsp118

Kaur, K., Salwi, S., McNew, K., Kumar, N., Millimet, H., Ravichandran, N., Tytus, K., Zhang, A. Y., Garrett Wood, A., Grimm, B., & Fairbrother, E. L. (2022). Medical student perspectives on the ethics of pelvic exams under anesthesia: A multi-institutional study. *Journal of Surgical Education, 79*(6), 1413–1421. https://doi.org/10.1016/j.jsurg.2022.05.015

Kearl, H. (2018). The facts behind the #MeToo movement: A national study on sexual harassment and assault. Stop Street Harassment. https://stopstreetharassment.org

Lunny, C., Taylor, D., Hoang, L., Wong, T., Razack, N., Buxton, J. A., Chernesky, M., & Garafalo, R. (2015). Self-collected versus clinician-collected sampling for chlamydia and gonorrhea: A systematic review and meta-analysis. *PLoS One, 10*(7), e0132776.

National Center for PTSD. (n.d.). *Sexual trauma: Information for women's medical providers*. US Department of Veterans Affairs.

Smith, S. G., Zhang, X., Basile, K. C., Merrick, M. T., Wang, J., Kresnow, M., & Chen, J. (2018). *The National Intimate Partner and Sexual Violence Survey (NISVS): 2015 data brief – updated release*. National Center for Injury Prevention and Control, Centers for Disease Control and Prevention.

US Department of Veterans Affairs, National Center for PTSD. (2021). Trauma and medical care. https://www.ptsd.va.gov/professional/treat/specific/trauma_medical.asp

Zuchelkowski, B. E., Eljamri, S., Stern, N. G., Varma, B., Arora, K. S., & Chang, J. C. (2022). Medical student attitudes on explicit informed consent for educational pelvic exams under anesthesia. *Journal of Surgical Education, 79*(3), 676–685. https://doi.org/10.1016/j.jsurg.2022.01.003

## Chapter 9

Singh Ospina, N., Phillips, K. A., Rodriguez-Gutierrez, R., Castaneda-Guarderas, A., Gionfriddo, M. R., Branda, M. E., Montori, V. M., & Thorsteinsdottir, B. (2019). Eliciting the patient's agenda: Secondary analysis of recorded clinical encounters. *Journal of General Internal Medicine, 34*(1), 36–40.

## Chapter 10

Andalibi, N., & Bowen, K. (2022). Internet-based information behavior after pregnancy loss: Interview study. *JMIR Formative Research, 6*(3), e32640. https://doi.org/10.2196/32640

Bellhouse, C., Temple-Smith, M., Kiropoulos, L., & Bilardi, J. (2024). The miscarriage circle of care: Towards leveraging online spaces for social support. *BMC Women's Health, 22*(1), 23.

Bellhouse, C., Temple-Smith, M., Watson, S., & Bilardi, J. (2024). Support sought and offered online for miscarriage: Content analysis of a Facebook miscarriage support group. *Psychology & Health, 38*(8), 1041–1058.

Cesare, N., Oladeji, O., Ferryman, K., Wijaya, D., & Hendricks-Muñoz, K. D. (2020). Discussions of miscarriage and preterm births on Twitter. *Paediatric and Perinatal Epidemiology, 34*(5), 544–552.

de Moel-Mandel, C., Donnelly, A., & Bugden, M. (2025). "Do you know what birth control actually does to your body?" Assessing contraceptive information on TikTok. *Perspectives on Sexual and Reproductive Health*, 358–367, https://doi.org/10.1111/psrh.70025

# References

Dubbelman, J., Ooms, J., Havgry, L., & Simonse, L. (2024). Communal load sharing of miscarriage experiences: Thematic analysis of social media community support. *Journal of Medical Internet Research, 26*, e56680.

Etactics. (2021). 50+ social media and healthcare statistics you need to know. https://etactics.com/blog/social-media-and-healthcare-statistics

Genetics in Medicine. (2021). Opportunities and pitfalls of social media research in rare genetic diseases: A systematic review. *Genetics in Medicine, 23*(12), 2238–2247. https://doi.org/10.1038/s41436-021-01255-w

Guttmacher Institute. (2025). Evidence-based sex education: The case for sustained federal support. https://www.guttmacher.org/fact-sheet/sex-education

Kbaier, D., Kane, A., McJury, M., & Kenny, I. (2024). Prevalence of health misinformation on social media—challenges and mitigation before, during, and beyond the COVID-19 pandemic: Scoping literature review. *Journal of Medical Internet Research, 26*, e38786.

Kirkpatrick, C. E., & Lawrie, L. L. (2024). TikTok as a source of health information and misinformation for young women in the United States: Survey study. *JMIR Infodemiology, 4*, e54663. https://doi.org/10.2196/54663

Lim, M. S. C., Molenaar, A., Brennan, L., Reid, M., & McCaffrey, T. (2022). Young adults' use of different social media platforms for health information: Insights from web-based conversations. *Journal of Medical Internet Research, 24*(1), e23656. https://doi.org/10.2196/23656

Media Market. (2025). *Social media in healthcare statistics and facts*. Author.

Merchant, R. M., South, E. C., & Lurie, N. (2021). Health information seeking behaviors on social media during the COVID-19 pandemic among American social networking site users: Survey study. *Journal of Medical Internet Research, 23*(6), e29802.

Mercier, R. J., Senter, K., Webster, R., & Riley Henderson, A. (2020). Instagram users' experiences of miscarriage. *Obstetrics & Gynecology, 135*(1), 166–173.

Mohamed, F., & Shoufan, A. (2024). Users' experience with health-related content on YouTube: An exploratory study. *BMC Public Health, 24*, 86. https://doi.org/10.1186/s12889-023-17585-5

Stanger-Hall, K. F., & Hall, D. W. (2011). Abstinence-only education and teen pregnancy rates: Why we need comprehensive sex education in the U.S. *PLoS One, 6*(10), e24658.

Villanti, A. C., Johnson, A. L., Ilakkuvan, V., Jacobs, M. A., Graham, A. L., & Rath, J. M. (2017). Social media use and access to digital technology in US young adults in 2016. *Journal of Medical Internet Research, 19*(6), e196. https://doi.org/10.2196/jmir.7303

## Chapter 11

Åsbring, P., & Närvänen, A. L. (2002). Women's experiences of stigma in relation to chronic fatigue syndrome and fibromyalgia. *Qualitative Health Research, 12*(2), 148–160.

Chen, E. H., Shofer, F. S., Dean, A. J., Hollander, J. E., Baxt, W. G., Robey, J. L., & Mills, A. M. (2008). Gender disparity in analgesic treatment of emergency department patients with acute abdominal pain. *Academic Emergency Medicine, 15*(5), 414–418.

Choshen-Hillel, S., Ishqer, A., Mahameed, F., Reiter, J., Gafter-Gvili, A., Millstein, T., ... & Gileles-Hillel, A. (2021). Physician and nurse pain estimations in the emergency department. *Proceedings of the National Academy of Sciences, 118*(33), e2101946118.

Hoffman, K. M., Trawalter, S., Axt, J. R., & Oliver, M. N. (2016). Racial bias in pain assessment and treatment recommendations, and false beliefs about biological differences between Blacks and Whites. *Proceedings of the National Academy of Sciences, 113*(16), 4296–4301.

Hollingshead, N. A., Matthias, M. S., Bair, M. J., & Hirsh, A. T. (2015). Impact of race and sex on pain management by medical trainees: A mixed methods pilot study of decision making and awareness of influence. *Pain Medicine, 16*(2), 280–290.

Kaler, A. (2006). Unreal women: Sex, gender, identity and the lived experience of vulvar pain. *Feminist Review, 82*(1), 50–75.

Kool, M. B., van Middendorp, H., Boeije, H. R., & Geenen, R. (2014). Understanding the lack of understanding: Invalidation from healthcare professionals and family members in patients with chronic fatigue syndrome and fibromyalgia. *Journal of Health Psychology, 19*(2), 240–251.

Moitra, E., Christopher, P. P., Harms, P. D., & Gaudiano, B. A. (2024). Medical gaslighting as a mechanism for medical trauma: Case studies and analysis. *Current Psychology, 43*(15), 13372–13380.

Ng, I. K. S., Lee, S. Z. L., Siantar, G. D., Tan, C., & Teo, D. B. (2024). Medical gaslighting: A new colloquialism. *The American Journal of Medicine, 137*(9), 823–826.

Nguyen, R. H. N., Turner, R. M., Rydell, S. A., MacLehose, R. F., & Harlow, B. L. (2013). Perceived stereotyping and seeking care for chronic vulvar pain. *Pain Medicine, 14*(10), 1461–1467.

Pletcher, M. J., Kertesz, S. G., Kohn, M. A., & Gonzales, R. (2008). Trends in opioid prescribing by race/ethnicity for patients seeking care in U.S. emergency departments. *JAMA, 299*(1), 70–78.

Rosenfeld, A. G. (2005). Treatment-seeking delay among women with acute myocardial infarction: Causes and consequences. *Circulation, 111*(4), 458–464.

Ruusuvuori, J., Poutiainen, S., Laakso, M., Raevaara, L., & Koskela, T. H. (2022). Interrupted opening statements in clinical encounters: A scoping review. *Patient Education and Counseling, 105*(7), 2122–2132.

Singh Ospina, N., Phillips, K. A., Rodriguez-Gutierrez, R., Castaneda-Guarderas, A., Gionfriddo, M. R., Branda, M. E., Montori, V. M., & Thorsteinsdottir, B. (2019). Eliciting the patient's agenda: Secondary analysis of recorded clinical encounters. *Journal of General Internal Medicine, 34*(1), 36–40.

Sun, T. Y., Hardin, J., Nieva, H. R., Natarajan, K., Cheng, R. F., Ryan, P., & Elhadad, N. (2023). Large-scale characterization of gender differences in diagnosis prevalence and time to diagnosis. *medRxiv.* https://doi.org/10.1101/2023.10.12.23296976

Westergaard, D., Moseley, P., Sørup, F. K. H., Baldi, P., & Brunak, S. (2019). Population-wide analysis of differences in disease progression patterns in men and women. *Nature Communications, 10*(1), 666.

## Chapter 17

Hatherall, B., Morris, J., Jamal, F., Sweeney, L., Wiggins, M., Kaur, I., Harden, A., & Renton, A. (2016). Timing of the initiation of antenatal care: An exploratory qualitative study of women and service providers in East London. *Social Science & Medicine, 154,* 97–104.

Moniz, M. H., Chang, T., Heisler, M., Admon, L. K., & Dalton, V. K. (2020). Out-of-pocket spending for maternity care among women with employer-based insurance, 2008–15. *Health Affairs, 39*(1), 18–23.

National Institute for Health and Care Excellence. (2021). *Antenatal care (NG201).* Author.

Simeonov, D., Mathews, T. J., & Curtin, S. C. (2021). National estimates of maternal healthcare costs in the United States, 2016–2018. *Medical Care, 59*(7), 635–642.

World Health Organization. (2023). *Trends in maternal mortality 2000 to 2020: Estimates by WHO, UNICEF, UNFPA, World Bank Group and the United Nations Population Division.* Author.